COLLINS GEM GUIDE ™

C000201250

Adriana Capadose

Nutrition Consultant: Jane F. Griffin

HarperCollins*Publishers*

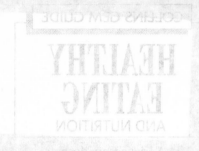

First published by HarperCollins Publishers 1991
© The Book Creation Company Ltd 1991
Reprint 10 9 8 7 6 5 4 3 2 1 0

ISBN 0 00 458991 2

Printed in Great Britain

Introduction

The Gem Guide to Healthy Eating and Nutrition is an easy-to-use pocket reference book. It provides an accessible and comprehensive guide to nutrition and diet.

The majority of the entries detail the content and nutritional value of basic foodstuffs, and how cooking, processing, storage or packaging effects their nutrient content.

The entries on nutrients explain their functions in the body, how much is required (recommended daily amount – RDA) and the foods and drinks in which they are found in significant amounts. Deficiency diseases and medical disorders related to nutrition are explained, as well as relevant biological terms. Cooking and processing terms are included. Some of the most important food additives are covered, but this subject requires a dictionary of its own and readers are recommended to consult the **Collins** *Gem Guide to Food Additives*.

The foods and drinks are entered under their common names, and not under manufacturers' brand names. The book is thoroughly cross-referenced, and cross-references appear in **bold lettering**.

Diet Through the Ages

Fossil evidence and anthropological studies show that early people were hunters and gatherers of food. They ate much more food containing fibre than we do today. Their predominantly vegetable diet meant that little of their protein came from animal foods, and they had a higher intake of certain minerals and vitamins. Their fat intake was low because what animal food they did eat came from wild animals with a higher lean-to-fat ratio than today's intensively farmed meat. Oil was not refined into a product but eaten as part of nuts and seeds. Sugars in the diet came from honey and fruits and there were no concentrated or refined products. Salt intakes were low, except among the communities living by the sea, who probably cooked with sea water. Much of the diet of early people fits current recommendations for a healthier diet.

Although they did not show signs of today's diet-related diseases, the hunter-gatherers were smaller in height with an average life expectancy of 30 years, and were far more active than we are today.

The nomadic lifestyle of the hunter-gatherers gradually declined with the development of agriculture some 10 000 years ago. In the more settled farming communities the diet began to change and with it came changes in health. Animals were reared specifically for food, and plants were cultivated to provide cereal crops. The diseases of affluence began to develop; those diseases caused by too much food rather than not enough – atherosclerosis, dental diseases, diabetes, gallstones, gout and obesity. The less well-off, however, continued to suffer from diseases caused by poor hygiene or lack of food.

Agricultural methods, and consequently the food supply, improved slowly over the centuries until the Agricultural and Industrial Revolutions of the 18th and 19th centuries. The great social and economic changes that resulted radically changed the diet. As the population grew and became urbanized, food was bought with wages rather than grown by and for each family, and cooking skills were lost as more food was bought from the bakeries, cook-houses and costermongers or barrow-boys, and the diet began to include imported foods.

From the 19th century through into the 20th, bread and potato consumption fell as that of fat and meat rose. The wide availability of foods meant that the diet was no longer dictated by supply but made up of foods of personal preference. By the 1960s, the diet contained as much meat, sugar, butter and cream as was wanted or could be afforded. Bread and potatoes (unless as chips and crisps) were mistakenly considered as nutritionally poor and fattening foods. The diet was high in fat, with a high proportion of saturated fatty acids, high in sugar and salt and low in starchy carbohydrates and dietary fibre.

Although there has been much publicity given to the need to change eating habits, the recommendations have, by and large, gone unheeded.

The diet in the United Kingdom still contains too much fat, sugar and salt and not enough dietary fibre and starchy carbohydrate. Our poor food choice is affecting our health.

Dietary Causes of Disease in Modern Britain

In Britain, the high intake of milk, butter and margarine and meat results in excessive intakes of fat with a high proportion of saturated fatty acids. Potatoes and flour (bread) are still staple foods, but they are often eaten with added fat; potatoes as chips or crisps, bread with butter or margarine and flour combined with butter, sugar and eggs to make puddings, cakes and biscuits. Meat remains a prized item in the diet and is still eaten in large amounts. With the exception of potatoes, the consumption of fruit and vegetables is low. Unlike many other countries, whole food has been replaced with processed and refined foods.

Obesity is not in itself a fatal disease, but one that increases the risk or severity of other illnesses. The more overweight a person is, the more likely they are to die at an earlier than average age. Being overweight increases the risk of developing several serious disorders, including high blood pressure (hypertension), which in turn causes stroke and heart disease, respiratory diseases, diabetes, gallstones, hernias and varicose veins. If you reach middle-age weighing 25 lbs extra, you can expect to die four years earlier than average, and Swedish research has shown that fat laid down around the abdomen carries more risk than fat around the hips and limbs. Of particular concern are overweight babies and children who may well carry their excess weight into adult life. Fat accumulates in the body when more food is eaten than the body needs for maintenance and physical activity. If energy intake equals energy output, body weight is steady; when energy intake exceeds energy output, body weight increases; when energy intake is less than energy output, body weight decreases.

Dental caries (tooth decay) is associated with excess sugar, especially when eaten frequently between meals. It causes toothache and, if neglected and allowed to develop, results in loss of teeth. Good dental hygiene and a controlled intake of sugar, preferably restricted to meal times, can be very effective in preventing dental caries.

Heart disease is the main cause of death in Britain, accounting for 25% of deaths every year. It is more common in men than women. Of particular concern are not the deaths in old age but the number of premature deaths from heart disease in men in the 45 to 64 age group.

The underlying problem in heart disease is atherosclerosis, which causes thickening of the arteries. Accumulation of fatty substances, particularly cholesterol, causes this thickening, but it is not so much the intake of cholesterol in the diet but the amount of cholesterol made by the body that is the problem. The more fat, particularly fat with a high saturated fatty acid content, in the diet, the more cholesterol is made. Some of the cholesterol is removed by high-density lipoproteins but the rest is deposited on the artery walls. These deposits build up, eventually blocking the flow of blood altogether. If this occurs in a blood vessel supplying the heart, it can cause a heart attack.

The risk of developing heart disease can be reduced by maintaining an acceptable body weight, eating less fat, particularly fat with a high proportion of saturated fatty acids, increasing dietary fibre intake by eating more fruit, vegetables and pulses, and possibly by eating more fatty fish. Non-dietary preventative actions include giving up smoking and taking more exercise. The contraceptive pill very slightly increases the risk of thrombosis after the age of 35. Users may consider changing to another form of contraception after discussion with their medical adviser.

High blood pressure or *hypertension* increases the risk of having a stroke or coronary thrombosis. These occur in both men and women and is a common cause of death in the under 60 age group. The causes are partly hereditary but also dietary. Dietary causes are probably obesity and a high intake of salt (sodium). Heavy drinking and use of the contraceptive pill also increase the risk of hypertension.

Diverticular disease is a common disease of the bowel or intestine. It is probably caused by a diet lacking in dietary fibre. Such a diet produces waste which is hard to push down through the intestines and the walls of the intestine thicken, making it even harder to evacuate the waste or faeces. The disease is characterized by pain, constipation with or without diarrhoea and bleeding. Piles or haemorrhoids may also be caused by diets low in dietary fibre, because the constipation resulting from such a diet causes straining and pressure on the veins around the anus and those in the legs.

Gallstones, more common in women than in men, are linked with dietary factors such as obesity, irregular meal patterns and a high sugar intake or a low dietary fibre intake.

Diabetes, in its two forms, affects 1% of the population. The first type of diabetes is not diet-related and requires treatment with insulin. The other, more common, type is diet-related and is a common complication of obesity. Surprisingly, it tends to be linked less with sugar intake than with fat intake. About 90% of all such cases are in middle-aged overweight people and the disease is often cured by nothing more complicated than a reducing diet.

Osteoporosis, a disease in which the bones become thin, brittle and prone to fracture, is very common in post-menopausal women. Although hormone replacement therapy appears the best preventative measure in older women, a good calcium and vitamin D intake, particularly in childhood and early adult life when the bones are accumulating calcium, is also important. Regular exercise also plays a preventative role.

Cancer is a disease that can take many different forms and there are many factors involved in causing them; some are hereditary, others are environmental. Dietary factors are involved in the initiation and promotion of cancer, but also in its prevention.

Initiators are the carcinogens in food, such as some moulds, nitrites and the compounds formed when food is smoked and pickled. Promoters in the diet include fat, salt and alcohol. High fat intakes are associated with cancer of the breast and bowel, high intakes of alcohol are associated with cancer of the oesophagus, mouth and larynx (the risk is greater among heavy-drinking smokers) and high salt intakes are associated with cancer of the stomach.

Protectors in the diet include vitamin A and C, hence the importance of including plenty of fresh fruit and vegetables in the diet. Consumption of complex carbohydrates (starch and dietary fibre) may have a protective effect against bowel cancer.

The Diet of Other Countries

The Southern Mediterranean countries (S. Italy, Spain and Greece) have less heart disease than the UK or the US, and their diets contain much less fat, particularly fat with a high proportion of saturated fatty acids.

When Italians eat meat, they eat mostly poultry, along with a large intake of vegetables (although not potatoes) and cereals in the form of pasta and bread. An Italian's fruit consumption is twice that of the average British person's. Milk, sugar and fats are not important components of the diet. That Italian food is fatty is a myth which probably arose because the fat is all visible, as olive oil (low in saturated fatty acid and high in mono-unsaturated fatty acids) and not hidden, as in the British diet.

The Spanish use pulses, particularly chickpeas and beans, which keep up the protein and dietary fibre intake without a high fat intake. Rice is used to make a little meat or fish go a long way, (paella), but bread is the mainstay of the diet. Olive oil, garlic and tomatoes are prominent, and pastry, pudding and cake, foods enjoyed often to excess by the British, are replaced by fresh fruit.

The cuisine of the Greeks is another that is based on olive oil and bread. Together they provide almost 60% of the total energy content of the Greek diet. Meat is eaten in small amounts, such as in stuffed peppers, and low fat yoghurts and goat's cheese (feta cheese) all contribute to keep the fat and saturated fatty acid content down. Fish is eaten as well as meat and the abundance of fruit, including citrus fruit, and the regular servings of salad boost the dietary fibre and vitamin C intakes.

The Indian diet is based on cereals (breads and rice) and pulses (lentils and beans), providing adequate protein, dietary fibre and vitamins without fat. Meat is used in small amounts, more as a flavouring, and as the animals are not reared intensively, the meat is leaner and contains less fat. Many Indians are vegetarian for religious reasons. Spices are used routinely and, although they have no specific role in healthy eating, they make vegetable dishes more varied and tasty. Ghee (clarified butter) has traditionally been used in Indian cooking, but vegetable oils are now becoming more popular.

In Chinese cooking, the raw materials are prepared in advance and then cooked at great speed, often in a wok. This preserves the nutrients and allows very little fat to be absorbed during the cooking. Steaming is another favourite method of cooking in China and this also minimizes nutrient losses. Cereals, such as rice, noodles and pasta, form the basis of the Chinese diet, which is about 80% vegetarian. As with Indian food, meat is only important as a flavouring in sauces, added together with plenty of lightly cooked vegetables to lend interest to the cereal portion of the meal. Dairy products are used very little but both salt and sugar are used frequently.

The Japanese diet relies on rice as the staple and meat is not eaten very much. Fish is more popular and is often eaten raw. Sugar and dairy foods are not used at all but the Japanese diet does have a very high salt content.

Eskimos enjoy good health and this has been linked to the amount of fish in the diet. Fatty fish contains a high proportion of two particular poly-unsaturated fatty acids which are believed to play a role in preventing heart disease.

A Balanced Diet

The nutrients that are the components of all foods are the same basic nutrients that all living tissue (including the human body) are made of. Food provides the energy and the essential nutrients for the body – carbohydrate (starch and dietary fibre), protein, fat, minerals, trace elements and vitamins. Most foods contain some, but not all, of the essential nutrients and it is necessary to eat as wide a variety of foods as possible to ensure that all the nutrient requirements are being met. Such a diet provides the material for growth and development in babies, children and adolescents, for the developing foetus and for milk production in the breast-feeding mother. It will provide the material for maintenance of the body and all bodily functions, and the energy for all movement and activity. Maintenance of health also depends on eating the right foods in the right amounts. Too much or too little food can lead to malnutrition. Not enough food causes starvation and mineral and vitamin deficiencies, too much causes obesity. The balance of the nutrients is also important in preventing the development of certain diseases, some of which are life-threatening. Too much sugar in the diet can cause dental decay and not enough dietary fibre has been linked with diseases of the bowel. Excessive intakes of fat are associated with heart disease and breast cancer and too much salt in the diet can lead to high blood pressure in susceptible people. A balanced, prudent or healthier diet is therefore one that takes all these considerations into account.

At present 42% of the energy in the average adult diet in the UK comes from fat, 41% from carbohydrate, 11% from protein and 6% from alcohol. The recommendation is that only 34% should come from fat, 50% should come from carbohydrate, 5% from alcohol and that protein should remain at 11%. The intake of saturated fatty acids should be reduced, as should the intake of sugar and salt, and the increased carbohydrate intake should be achieved by eating more and varied complex or starchy carbohydrates rich in dietary fibre.

In terms of food in the diet these recommendations can be followed in this way: **1.** Eat generous amounts at each meal of bread, pasta, potatoes, breakfast cereals or other cereals, choosing wholegrain cereals where possible. **2.** Eat three or more servings a day of fresh fruit and vegetables. **3.** Eat two or more servings a day of lean meat, poultry, (shellfish, fish, pulses—peas, beans or lentils—offal) or eggs. **4.** Reduce the amount of full milk or take semi-skimmed or skimmed milk (at least half a pint a day), and low fat yoghurt or reduced fat cheese. **5.** Butter, margarine and vegetable oils should be used only sparingly. A low fat spread could be used as an alternative. **6.** Sugar, sweets, biscuits and soft drinks containing sugar should be used only sparingly. **7.** No more alcohol than the recommended maximum of 21 units a week for men and 14 units a week for women should be consumed. A unit is equivalent to a single shot of spirits, a glass of wine or half a pint of ordinary beer.

absorption The process by which the **nutrients** and **micronutrients** from food are passed across the wall of the gut into the bloodstream after digestion.

acacia gum The thick, sticky gum that collects and dries on the stem and branches of certain varieties of acacia tree. The gum is used as a food **additive** to thicken sweets, jellies and glazes and to maintain the foam on beer and soft drinks.

acceptable weight The weight or range of weights considered acceptable for a person according to their age, height and sex. For a table of acceptable weights see APPENDIX I, LOSING AND GAINING WEIGHT.

acetic acid An acid found in vinegar. It is added to pickles and sauces as a preservative and acidifier. It is also produced in the body and is involved in energy release, and the fermentation of dietary fibre in the intestines.

acid A substance that has a **pH** of less than 7. Very strong acids are corrosive and dangerous. Many foods contain mild acids, e.g. **citric acid** in citrus fruit and **acetic acid** in vinegar. The stomach secretes acidic digestive juices to help break down foods. If the body's pH balance, or **acid-base balance**, is disturbed by an excess of acidic substances, a condition known as **acidosis** may occur. See also **alkali**.

acid-base balance The balance of **acids** and **alkalis** in the body. The blood has a **pH** of 7.35–7.45, and this fine balance is maintained by the excretion of excess acids or alkalis, via the kidneys, in the urine and acid breathed out through the lungs. The urine of omnivores is usually slightly acid; vegetarians have neutral urine, neither acid or alkali; and carnivores have the most acid urine. Fruits and vegetables are alkali-producing foods, although they often have an acidic taste because of the presence of acids such as **citric acid**, **oxalic acid** and tartaric acid. The stomach contents are acid because of the presence of hydrochloric acid in the gastric juices. The body can deal with the relative acidity and alkalinity of foods and no attention need be paid to balancing acidity and alkalinity in the diet.

acidosis A condition in which the **pH** of the body fluids is very low, i.e. they are very acid. Acidosis is caused by a dramatic increase in acidity or a draining of alkalines in the body fluids. It may occur as a result of diabetes, liver diseases, kidney disorders, severe diarrhoea or excessive physical exertion. Acidosis is characterized by rapid breathing, tiredness and possibly vomiting and should be treated by a doctor.

acne A skin disorder common among teenagers and may occur as one of the symptoms of premenstrual syndrome. Acne affects the hair and sweat glands on the face, neck and upper body. The glands become inflamed and form clusters of small pustules. Although avoidance of fatty food, sweets and chocolate are often recommended, their role in causing acne has not been proven. High intakes of **vitamin A** and **zinc** have been used in the treatment of acne.

additive   A natural or artificial substance that manufacturers add to foods to improve their appearance, consistency and palatability and to extend their shelf-life and to aid processing methods. Food additives include: **preservatives**, **artificial colourings** and **flavourings**, **sweeteners**, anti-caking agents, anti-foaming agents, **antioxidants**, bleaching agents, emulsifiers, flavour enhancers, gelling agents, stabilizers and thickeners. Some of these substances may cause allergic reactions, such as aggravating eczema, provoking **asthma** attacks and causing **hyperactivity**.

Under food labelling regulations all food additives must be listed on food labels by type and chemical name or number. Labels should always be checked closely, because a product labelled 'no artificial preservatives' may well contain other additives and foods labelled 'no artificial additives' may contain natural additives.

adipose tissue   The collection of fat cells that makes up the body's store of **fat**. An excess accumulation of adipose tissue gives rise to **overweight** and **obesity**. See also APPENDIX I, LOSING AND GAINING WEIGHT.

adrenal gland A small gland situated above each kidney. The adrenal gland secretes a number of hormones, including adrenaline. Adrenaline is released at times of stress. It quickens the heart and breathing rate, raises the **blood glucose** level, increases the circulation of blood to the muscles and improves the efficiency with which the muscles use blood glucose. These physiological changes prepare the body for the demands of excessive physical activity. If the release of adrenaline is not accompanied by physical exertion, it may cause 'jitteriness', fluttering of the heart, giddiness and, in extreme cases, nausea and fainting. The correct functioning of the adrenal gland requires a good intake of **vitamin C** and **pantothenic acid**. Excessive adrenal activity at times of acute stress may deplete the body's levels of these vitamins. See also **stress**.

adzuki bean The red-brown seed of the Asian adzuki plant, a **pulse**. Adzuki beans provide **protein**, **starch**, **dietary fibre**, some **sugars** and have an energy value of 142 kcal/100 g (boiled). They also contain **calcium**, **thiamin**, **riboflavin** and **niacin**, and some **iron**, **manganese**, **molybdenum** and **carotene**. Like other pulses, adzuki beans contain small amounts of **phytic acid** and **lectins**, and should be thoroughly cooked to destroy these substances.

aflatoxin A toxic substance produced by a fungus (*Aspergillus flavus*). Aflatoxins, which can cause liver diseases, are formed by moulds that may develop on nuts and cereals stored in a warm, moist atmosphere. They can usually be detected by a white bloom on nuts or by a musty taste.

agar   A structural **polysaccharide** extracted from seaweed that contributes to **dietary fibre**. Agar is used as a gelling agent and a stabilizer. It is acceptable to vegans because it is not extracted from animals and is a useful alternative to **gelatin**.

alcohol   The intoxicating, colourless liquid derived from the **fermentation** of **sugars**. Alcohol is found in spirits, wine, beer, cider and other intoxicating drinks. A healthy adult can consume 20 to 30 ml of alcohol a day without damaging their health. However, the damage to health of excessive alcohol intake cannot be overestimated. In the short term, the feeling of intoxication is accompanied by distorted perception and impaired judgement, and is usually followed by a headache and dehydration. Alcohol and alcoholic drinks have high energy values, but have virtually no nutritional values and may contribute to weight gain. Frequent excessive drinking is often accompanied by a reduction in food intake, which may lead to mineral and vitamin deficiencies. Alcohol raises the blood pressure, puts a strain on the kidneys and causes damage to the liver. Over long periods, this may cause **cirrhosis** of the liver, or other liver complaints. Alcohol interferes with the absorption of **zinc**, **magnesium**, **potassium**,

vitamin C, thiamin, folic acid and **vitamin K**, and it increases the absorption of toxic lead. In the long term, alcohol can cause brain damage and may increase susceptibility to some forms of cancer. Frequent excessive drinking can cause alcohol dependency (alcoholism). Long-term alcohol addiction or even one isolated massive intake of alcohol can be fatal. It is extremely damaging to the foetus and may cause malformations, slow development and even brain damage in the foetus, and should be cut out altogether during pregnancy.

alcohol-free drink   Any drink that does not contain more than 0.05% alcohol by volume. Alcohol-free and de-alcoholized drinks must declare the alcohol content on the label. Drinks labelled 'low alcohol' must contain no more than 1.2% alcohol by volume. Drinks labelled 'reduced alcohol' do not have to conform to a set standard alcohol content.

ale   A kind of **beer** not flavoured with hops. There are three different types of ale: brown, pale or light and strong ale. They contain 2.5, 3.5 and 7% alcohol by volume, respectively. Strong ale has almost twice the energy value (72 kcal/100 g) of brown ale (28 kcal/100 g) and pale ale (32 kcal/100 g). All ales provide **folic acid**, with strong ale containing twice as much as brown and pale ale.

alfalfa   The highly nutritious seeds of a plant used as fodder for animals. Alfalfa seeds can be soaked for several days to form sprouts, which are a good source of minerals and vitamins. They contain small amounts of **protein** and **dietary fibre**, and have an energy value of 36 kcal/100 g (soaked). Alfalfa sprouts provide **iron**, **calcium**, **potassium**, **phosphorus**, **magnesium**, **carotene**, **thiamin**, **niacin**, **vitamin C**, **vitamin D**, **vitamin E** and **vitamin K**, and are one of the few plant sources of **vitamin B$_{12}$**. They have a mild **diruetic** effect.

alga A general name for very simple forms of plant life that grow in fresh or salt water or on moist ground. Certain aquatic alga, such as **kelp** and **spirulina**, are valued, particularly by vegetarians and vegans, for their nutritional content.

alginate A **polysaccharide** gel with similar properties to **edible gums** (i.e. it is a form of **dietary fibre**). Alginate is obtained from **kelp**, and is used commercially as an emulsifier, thickener, stabilizer and gelling agent in a variety of foods, including instant puddings, ice cream and processed cheese.

alkali (also called **base**) A substance that has a **pH** of more than 7. Some of the digestive juices that break down foods are mild alkalis, e.g. the juices secreted by the pancreas. A healthy body maintains a delicate **acid-base balance**. If the body's pH balance is disturbed by an excess of alkalinity, an unusual condition known as alkalosis may occur. Alkalosis may be caused by repeated vomiting or excessive urination, and its symptoms include weakness and muscle cramps. It should be treated by a doctor. See also **acid**.

allergy (food) A hypersensitive reaction to a substance in the diet that causes the body's immune system to release **histamine**. Many people suffer from food allergies, which may cause a harmless and short-lived rash (e.g. strawberry rash, caused by eating strawberries) or an inability to digest certain foods correctly (e.g. cows' milk and milk products), to violent vomiting. Other common symptoms of food allergies are **eczema** and **urticaria**, **oedema**, headaches, migraines, congestion in the nose and sinuses, **asthma**, heart palpitations, and various digestive complaints (such as diarrhoea, vomiting, constipation and flatulence) and nervous disorders (such as **hyperactivity** and clumsiness). In some cases, the immune system may gradually develop a tolerance to the allergen (the allergy-inducing substance), but in most cases the allergen must be identified by a slow process of elimination and then avoided. Confirmation of a food allergy should be carried out by a doctor or dietitian. Some common food allergens include: cows' milk and milk products, eggs, wheat, maize, rye, chocolate, fish, oranges, tomatoes, pork and beef. In many cases, these allergens may be replaced by alternative foods, e.g. cows' milk with goats' milk or ewes' milk. Two food additives that commonly cause allergies are

tartrazine (E102) and benzoic acid (E210), a pre-servative.

allspice The seeds of a tropical American tree that are dried and used whole or ground to add flavour to foods such as patés, sausages and meat pies. The name is derived from the fact that all-spice tastes like a combination of cinnamon, cloves and nutmeg. Allspice is used in such small quantities that its nutritional properties are negli-gible.

almond The nut-like seed of a small tree of West Asian origin, eaten whole as a nut or used in cook-ing for its distinctive flavour. Almonds are rich in **fat** with a high proportion of **polyunsaturated fatty acid**, they provide **protein**, **dietary fibre** and some **sugars**, and have an energy value of 565 kcal/100 g. They are rich in **potassium**, **phosphorus**, **vitamin E** and **lecithin**, and also contain some **manganese**, **zinc**, **niacin** and **folic acid**. Although they contain **calcium**, **iron** and **magnesium**, little is absorbed because of the presence of **oxalic** and **phytic acid**. Almonds may be served as a salted snack, in which case they have a very high **sodium** content.

almond paste A smooth, rich, pale-yellow coloured paste traditionally made with ground **almonds**, icing sugar and eggs. Almond paste pro-vides the **nutrients** and **micronutrients** associated with almonds and eggs and has an energy value of 443 kcal/100 g. Manufactured almond paste may not be made with eggs, and may also contain artificial colourings, flavourings and preservatives.

aluminium   A metallic element, not known to be essential to humans, although it is present in the body and in food (e.g. lentils, rice and tea). Aluminium may also be ingested from foods cooked in aluminium pans, prepared using aluminium utensils or stored in aluminium foil. It is present in some of the food additives that are commonly used in processed cheese, baking powder and table salt. Excesses of aluminium are normally expelled by the bowels. However, research suggests that very high levels of aluminium are not readily excreted by the body, and that they may cause the brain to become more vulnerable to toxic substances. This has been linked with failing memory and **Alzheimer's disease**.

Alzheimer's disease   A disease that impairs the memory, especially recent memory, and reduces the ability to 'register' new memories. The symptoms are the same as those displayed by elderly people suffering from senile dementia, but Alzheimer's disease can occur at any age. The exact causes of the disease are not known, and it should be diagnosed and treated by a doctor. Aluminium, although not thought to be an essential nutrient, has been shown to accumulate in the brain and it may have an involvement in this disease.

amino acid One of a number of organic compounds that are the building blocks of **proteins**. There are 20 amino acids in the human body: 12 non-essential (i.e. they can be synthesized by the body), alanine, aspartic acid, arginine, cysteine, glutamic acid, glycine, histidine, hydroxyproline, ornithine, proline, serine and tyrosine; 8 essential (i.e. they cannot be synthesized by the body, and must be obtained from the diet), isoleucine, leucine, lysine, methionine, phenylalanine, threonine, tryptophan and valine. Amino acids are used to synthesize all the body proteins, including **enzymes** and hormones, and are vital for growth and health.

In order to build up protein efficiently in the body, all the essential amino acids must be provided by the diet, and the easiest way of ensuring this is to eat foods that are good sources of protein (e.g. animal foods, milk and milk products, wholegrain cereals, pulses, nuts and seeds). In general, animal sources of protein contain all the essential amino acids in the proportions required by the body. Plant sources may be lacking in one particular amino acid, which reduces the usefulness of the entire protein content of the food. The amino acid that is present in small quantities is known as the limiting amino acid. Strict **vegans** should ensure that they combine foods that have different limiting amino acids to make up the full complement of essential amino acids, such as a combination of pulses and cereals (e.g. baked beans on wholemeal toast).

anaemia The general name for a number of disorders affecting either the number or shape and functioning of red **blood cells**. A reduction in the number of these cells, or a malformation, reduces the supply of oxygen to the muscles, the brain and other organs. The symptoms of all forms of anaemia are fatigue, paleness, shortness of breath, heart palpitations, poor appetite, dizziness and even fainting.

The most common form of anaemia is iron-deficiency anaemia. **Iron** is a vital part of red blood cells and if the dietary intake of iron is inadequate, or if there are excessive losses of blood (through injury or heavy menstruation), the red blood cells develop incorrectly and cause anaemia. The body's requirement for iron is increased during pregnancy and lactation, and iron deficiency anaemia is common at these times. It can be treated with large doses of iron, sometimes with supplements of **vitamin C** and **copper**. **Protein** is also vital to the correct formation of red blood cells, and people with a susceptibility to anaemia should ensure that their protein intake is adequate (red meats provide protein and are rich in iron). Other forms of anaemia may be caused by deficiencies of other vitamins associated with the formation of red blood cells, e.g. **vitamin B_{12}, folic acid, vitamin E** and **vitamin B_6**. If the symptoms are severe or prolonged medical advice and diagnosis should be sought.

anchovy Tiny, marine, fatty fish of the herring

family, usually canned in vegetable oil. Anchovies are usually eaten in fairly small quantities to add flavour to dishes. They provide **protein** and **fat**, and have an energy value of 143 kcal/100 g. Anchovies also contain **potassium**, **phosphorus**, **vitamin B₁₂** and some **calcium**, **zinc** and **niacin**. They have a very high **sodium** content.

angelica The candied, aromatic stem of a tall, white-flowered plant. Angelica is used to add flavour and as a garnish in sweet dishes. It is used in such small quantities that its nutritional properties are virtually negligible. It is very high in **sugars** and has an energy value of 321 kcal/100 g.

aniseed The highly flavoured, aromatic seeds of the Mediterranean anise plant. Aniseed is used for its pleasant liquorice flavour in confectionery, desserts and spirits. It is used in very small quantities and its nutritional properties are negligible. Aniseed infusions are sometimes used to relieve flatulence.

anorexia nervosa A psychological disorder characterized by an obsession with body weight and weight loss. Anorexia nervosa may have a number of psychological causes, and may develop in a person of either sex and of any age, but it most often occurs among adolescent girls and young women. It is characterized by a dissatisfaction with personal appearance, a determination to lose weight and a refusal to eat. Some anorexics may be preoccupied with food and may not actually have any loss of appetite. Many indulge in self-induced vomiting and laxative abuse. Anorexia nervosa causes dramatic weight loss, and sufferers display the symptoms of malnutrition, including multiple vitamin and mineral deficiencies. Mood swings, bouts of listlessness followed by hyperactivity, and amenorrhoea (absence of menstruation) in women are common features. Anorexia nervosa is a potentially fatal disorder and sufferers must seek psychiatric treatment. See also **bulimia nervosa**.

antibiotics Drugs used medicinally to destroy microorganisms, e.g. bacteria, that cause infections and infectious diseases. Antibiotics are also used in animals and consequently people who have become allergic to antibiotics may react to the small amounts in meat and offal. Antibiotics are known to alter the normal growth of microorganisms in the gut and can cause diarrhoea, which if prolonged can lead to malnutrition. Some antibiotics decrease the body's ability to absorb vitamins and minerals.

antioxidant A substance used in **fats** and **oils**, and thereby in foods containing them, to delay, retard or prevent the development of rancidity or other flavour deterioration due to oxidation. Fats and oils, when they come into contact with oxygen in the air, are oxidized and this makes them go rancid, giving them an 'off' flavour and often causing sickness if eaten. Antioxidants are used in food products such as butter, margarine, meat products, cakes, biscuits and pastry. Antioxidants are also added to non-fat foods, such as cut fruit to prevent discoloration, again caused by oxidation. **Vitamin E** and **vitamin C** have antioxidant functions in the body and they are also used commercially. Manufacturers also use a number of artificial substances that may cause allergies in some people. Antioxidants as food additives are assigned the E numbers E220-E330.

antivitamin A substance that destroys or interferes with the absorption of vitamins. Antivitamins include toxic substances, some drugs and alcohol. Excesses of certain minerals and excesses of some vitamins may themselves act as antivitamins.

apple The fruit of the apple tree, widely cultivated in temperate climates, with thin green, yellow or red skin, crisp white flesh and a bitter core containing dark seeds. There are many varieties of eating and cooking apple. Their nutritional properties are all similar they contain **sugars** and some **dietary fibre** (including **pectin**). Cooking apples contain less sugar than eating apples and their energy value is correspondingly lower at 37 kcal/100 g. Eating apples have an energy value of 46 kcal/100 g. Apples also provide some **potassium**, **vitamin C** and **folic acid**. Cooking apples have a higher vitamin C content, but much

of the vitamin C content is lost when apples are
peeled. There are few losses of vitamins when
apples are stewed or baked. Dried apples provide
proportionally more sugar, dietary fibre, potassium and folic acid by weight, but they contain
hardly any vitamin C. Apple juice contains **sugars**
and small amounts of **vitamin C** and **folic acid**, and
has an energy value of 39 kcal/100 ml. See also
fruit juices.

apple juice See **apple**.

apricot A small fruit with thin, smooth orange
skin and soft, sweet flesh around a hard stone.
Apricots contain **sugars**, some **dietary fibre**, a
small amount of **protein** and have an energy value
of 28 kcal/100 g. They are a good source of **carotene**, and also provide **potassium**, and some
copper, **vitamin C** and **folic acid**. Only the folic acid
content is seriously depleted if apricots are stewed.
Dried apricots provide proportionately more
sugars and dietary fibre by weight, and have an
energy value of 186 kcal/100 g. They are a rich
source of carotene and a good source of folic acid,
but they contain no vitamin C. Again the folic
acid content is seriously depleted if dried apricots
are stewed. Canned apricots contain the same
micronutrients as fresh apricots, but some of the
vitamin C is lost; further losses of vitamin C occur
if they are stored for a longtime. Apricots canned
in syrup have an energy value of 107 kcal/100 g.

arrowroot The easily digested **starch** extracted

from the root of a plant of West Indian origin. Arrowroot is used in the home and by manufacturers to thicken food. It is very high in starch, has an energy value of 355 kcal/100 g, but does not contain significant amounts of any **micronutrients**.

arsenic A metallic element that is essential for growth in some animals and may be essential in humans, but its functions – if any – are not yet known. Arsenic is highly toxic in excess, but the average daily intake is well within safe limits.

arthritis A disease that affects the joints, causing painful inflammation and stiffness. There are two kinds of arthritis: rheumatoid arthritis and **osteoarthritis**. Rheumatoid arthritis causes painful stiffness and inflammation of the joints, and may be accompanied by muscular stiffness. It can affect the sufferer's general health, causing loss of appetite and sickness, and it may be accompanied by fever and **anaemia**. The exact causes of arthritis are not known, but dietary factors may be involved. Supplements of **calcium**, **niacin** and **vitamin C** may help to relieve the symptoms.

artificial colouring Food additives used by manufacturers to enhance the colour and appearance of foods. There are some 45 colourings permitted in the UK, of which just under half are artificial, the rest being natural (e.g. turmeric and saffron). Artificial colourings may cause allergic reactions in some people, such as rashes, breath-

17

ing difficulties and **hyperactivity**. Shoppers trying to avoid foods that have been treated with artificial colourings should check the ingredients on the label, and look for foods labelled 'free of artificial colours'.

artificial flavour   Food additives used by manufacturers to give flavour to foods. Many foods are flavoured with natural ingredients, but there are chemical substances which mimic natural flavours, and are easier to use and cheaper than natural sources. Artificial flavours are less likely to cause an allergic response than **artificial colours**, although many hyperactive children are recommended to avoid them. Shoppers trying to avoid foods that contain artificial flavours should check the ingredients on the label, and look for foods labelled 'free of artificial flavours'.

ascorbic acid   The chemical name for **vitamin C**.

asparagus   The succulent stem and leaves of the young asparagus plant. There are many different varieties of asparagus and it may be eaten at different stages of growth. In general, it has a high water content and provides only small amounts of **protein**, **sugars** and **dietary fibre**, and has an energy value of 18 kcal/100 g (boiled). It also contains some **copper**, **carotene**, **vitamin C**, **vitamin E** and **folic acid**. Almost all of the vitamin C content is lost in canned asparagus, which also contain added salt and have a high **sodium** content. If asparagus is served with vinaigrette or butter, the energy value is greatly increased.

aspartame An intense **sweetener** made up of two **amino acids**, phenylalanine and aspartic acid. It has virtually no energy value, but is 200 times sweeter than **sucrose**. Aspartame is the sweetener used in Nutrasweet and Canderel. It is used commercially to make low-calorie soft drinks, cordials and desserts, including yoghurts. It is available as a table sweetener in liquid and tablet form. Aspartame and products in which it has been used should not be eaten by people suffering from phenylketonuria (an inherited disease affecting the metabolism of the essential amino acid phenylalanine).

aspic A savoury jelly made from meat or fish stock, and used as a mould for cold dishes. Stock contains some of the protein and micronutrients of the meat or fish from which it is derived. It is usually salty and, therefore, has a high **sodium** content. Manufactured aspic may contain colourings, flavourings, preservatives and other additives.

assimilation The process by which nutrients and micronutrients in food are used by the body. Food is broken down in the mouth, stomach and intestines, and the individual nutrients and micronutrients are assimilated (used) by the tissues to carry out all the processes of metabolism.

The efficient assimilation of some micronutrients may depend on the presence of others or may be interrupted by excesses or deficiencies of others, e.g. a low intake of biotin reduces the body's ability to assimilate folic acid and vitamin B_{12}, the presence of vitamin D aids calcium metabolism.

asthma A respiratory disorder characterized by difficulty in breathing, wheezing and a feeling of constriction in the chest. Asthma may be hereditary and attacks can be caused by physical exertion, allergies and stress. Eggs, cheese, milk, nuts, seafood and some food additives (particularly colouring and preservatives) are the most common food causes.

atherosclerosis Thickening of the artery walls. Atherosclerosis is caused by a build-up of fatty substances, including **cholesterol**, in the artery walls. These deposits narrow the blood vessel and restrict the flow of blood. This may cause small blood clots, which then become incorporated in the artery wall, further narrowing the vessel. Narrowing can occur anywhere in the body, but if it is in arteries supplying the heart it can cause **coronary heart disease** and in the brain, **stroke**. The risk of developing atherosclerosis can be lowered by reducing the amount of **fat** in the diet, particularly fat with a high proportion of **saturated fatty acids**, and ensuring that the fat that is eaten contains a high proportion of **polyunsaturated fatty acids**.

aubergine (also called **eggplant**)   The fruit of a tropical Asian plant with thin, tough, glossy dark purple skin and pithy whitish flesh. Aubergines provide **sugars**, **dietary fibre**, small amounts of **protein** and **starch**, and have an energy value of 14 kcal/100 g. They also contain small amounts of **vitamin C** and **folic acid**. When aubergines are fried they absorb large amounts of oil, which increases the energy value. Frying also destroys their vitamin C content.

avocado pear   The pear-shaped fruit of a tropical tree of American origin, with smooth green or knobbly black skin and smooth yellow flesh around a large brown seed. Unusually for a fruit, avocado pears contain moderate amounts of **fat**, with a high proportion of **unsaturated fatty acid**. They also contain some **protein**, small amounts of **sugars** and **dietary fibre**, and have an energy value of 223 kcal/100 g. Avocado pears also provide **potassium**, **folic acid** and **biotin**, and some **carotene** and **vitamin C**. Compared to other fruits, avocado pears have a high energy value, and they are usually served with salad dressings, which further adds to the energy value.

bacon   Pig meat (usually from the back and sides of the animal) that has been cured and may also be smoked. Bacon provides **protein** and has a high **fat** content, and a correspondingly high energy value. The proportion of fat varies according to the cut, and the energy value can be lowered by trimming

21

some of the visible fat before or after cooking. Grilled lean bacon has an energy value of 147 kcal/100 g and fried streaky bacon has an energy value of 496 kcal/100 g. It also provides **potassium**, **phosphorus** and **niacin**, and some **iron**, **zinc**, **thiamin**, **vitamin B₆**, **pantothenic** acid and **biotin**. All bacon is salted, and has a very high **sodium** content. Bacon is usually fried or grilled; if it is grilled it will have less fat and therefore a lower energy value than if it is fried. None of the vitamins are seriously depleted when bacon is cooked. Bacon contains **nitrates** and **nitrites** added during curing.

B complex vitamins A group of water-soluble vitamins. The B complex vitamins are: **thiamin** (vitamin B₁), **riboflavin** (vitamin B₂), **niacin** (vitamin B₃), **pantothenic acid** (vitamin B₅), **vitamin B₆** (pyridoxine), **vitamin B₁₂**, **biotin** (vitamin H) and **folic acid**. Each vitamin has specific functions in the body, including growth and development in the young, energy release from nutrients, the maintenance of healthy skin and blood and the correct functioning of the nervous and digestive systems. These vitamins often occur together in the same foods, although different foods provide them in different proportions. Most of them are found in milk, cheese, liver, pulses, green vegetables, wholegrain cereals and brewer's yeast (vitamin B₁₂ is exceptional in that it is found in few plant sources).

There are different **RDAs** for each of the B complex vitamins, and the deficiency symptoms for each of them are also specific, but, because they are found together, a deficiency of only one of these vitamins is unlikely to occur. A deficiency of all B complex vitamins causes general poor condition, and digestive, nervous and skin complaints. Excesses of B complex vitamins are excreted in the urine. The vitamins that are not included in the B complex are the fat-soluble vitamins (vitamin A, vitamin D, vitamin E and vitamin K) and vitamin C, another water-soluble vitamin.

bacteria Microscopic organisms present in the body and in almost every form of food. Some forms of bacteria are harmful to people, but those that are found in the intestine (the intestinal flora) are essential to health because they synthesize **vitamin K** and **biotin**, and help break down food. Antibiotic drugs may destroy this bacteria, but they can be replaced by eating live yoghurt. If the bacteria in food are not destroyed by heat treatment (sterilization, pasteurization, ultra heat treatment or cooking) or chemical preservatives, and if conditions are conducive to their reproduction (they reproduce in warm and moist conditions and their reproduction is inhibited by drying or refrigeration), they can damage food and they may cause food poisoning. The risks of food poisoning can be minimized by respecting the sell-by dates on foods, following the manufacturer's storage instructions and thorough cooking.

baked bean A baked **haricot bean** canned in tomato sauce. Baked beans, including the tomato sauce, provide **protein**, **starch**, **dietary fibre** and **sugars**, and have an energy value of 64 kcal/100 g. They also contain **iron** and **manganese**, and some **niacin**, **vitamin E** and **folic acid**. They have a high **sodium** content, and may contain added sugar, colourings and flavourings.

baking A method of cooking in the oven, using high temperatures but no water or fat (other than fat that may be an ingredient of foods being baked). No vitamins are lost by **leaching** into cooking water, but some vitamins (**riboflavin**, **thiamin** and **vitamin C**) may be destroyed or depleted by the high temperatures. If **baking powder** is used to make doughs rise, the combination of high temperatures and alkaline conditions destroys riboflavin, **vitamin B₁₂ and pantothenic acid**.

baking powder A substitute for **yeast** used as a raising agent in baking cakes and bread. Baking powder usually contains sodium bicarbonate, which is alkaline, and small amounts of cream of tartar, which is acidic. At high temperatures, the reaction between these two ingredients releases carbon dioxide gas, which forms tiny bubbles within the dough, causing it to rise and giving it a light, spongy texture when cooked. Baking powder is predominantly an alkaline preparation, and it may cause losses of some micronutrients that are destroyed by high temperatures in alkaline conditions, e.g. **riboflavin, vitamin B$_{12}$ and pantothenic acid**.

balanced diet   See the introductory chapter, A BALANCED DIET.

bamboo shoot   The crisp, young stem of bamboo grass. Bamboo shoots provide **dietary fibre**, some **sugars** and **protein**, and have an energy value of 18 kcal/100 g. They also contain some **vitamin C** and **folic acid**. If they are canned, much of the vitamin C and folic acid contents are lost, and they may also contain added salt and have a high **sodium** content.

banana   The crescent-shaped fruit of a small, tropical palm-like tree with thick yellow skin and sweet, starchy off-white flesh. Bananas provide **sugars**, **starch** and **dietary fibre**, and small amounts of **protein**. They have an energy value of 79 kcal/100 g and also contain **potassium** and **folic acid**, and some **carotene** and **vitamin B$_6$**.

barbecuing   A method of cooking, usually meat or fish, over an open flame or hot coals. Barbecuing exposes the outside of the food to high temperatures (over 100°C) and may cause slight losses of vitamins that are unstable at high temperatures, e.g. **thiamin** and **pantothenic acid**. Other vitamins and minerals, e.g. **potassium**, may be **leached** into the juices that escape from food during cooking. Barbecuing lowers the fat content and energy value as fat drips out under the intense heat.

barley A cereal used commercially to make beer and whisky, and as an ingredient of soups and stews. Barley provides **starch** and small amounts of **protein**, and has an energy value of 327 kcal/100 g. It also contains **phosphorus**, **manganese**, **zinc**, **sulphur**, **molybdenum**, **niacin**, **vitamin E**, **vitamin B₆**, **folic acid** and **pantothenic acid**. Barley is usually available for domestic use as **pearl barley**.

barley water A soft drink traditionally made from **pearl barley** boiled in water and flavoured with orange or lemon juice. Manufactured barley water contains 2% **starch** but no other nutrients in significant amounts, and it may contain colouring and flavouring.

basal metabolic rate (BMR) The amount of energy required by the resting body to carry out metabolic processes, and to maintain the normal body temperature. BMR is higher in babies and growing children in relation to body size than adults, and drops when full height and sexual maturity are reached, declining gradually throughout adult life. Men have a slightly higher BMR than women, and conditions, such as external temperature, pregnancy, stress, illness or injury, may change the BMR.

base See **alkali**.

basil The aromatic leaves of a Eurasian plant used fresh or dried, whole or powdered as a herb. Basil is used in such small quantities that its nutritional properties are negligible.

bay The leaves of a species of Mediterranean laurel tree, used fresh or dried to give flavour to food. Bay leaves are not eaten but soaked in foods during cooking to give off flavour.

bean The seed or young seed pod of certain **pulses**. The energy values and nutritional properties of different kinds of bean vary. In general, those that are eaten as mature seeds (e.g. **adzuki bean**, **broad bean**, **butter bean**, **haricot bean**, **kidney bean**, **mung bean**, and **soya bean**) have higher energy values and are more nutritious than those that are eaten as pods (e.g. **French bean** and **runner bean**).

beansprout A soya bean that has been soaked for several days to produce a sprout. Beansprouts provide **protein**, **sugars** and **dietary fibre**, and have an energy value of 9 kcal/100 g. They also contain **calcium**, **iron**, **manganese**, **molybdenum**, **riboflavin**, **vitamin B$_6$**, **vitamin C**, **vitamin E** and **vitamin K**. If they are canned, much of the vitamin C content is lost, and they may contain added salt and have a high **sodium** content.

beef The meat of various bovine animals, especially the cow. The energy value and nutritional properties of beef vary according to the cut. In general it provides **protein** and **fat** with a high proportion of **saturated fatty acid** (the fat content and corresponding energy value can be reduced by trimming visible fat before or after cooking). Beef is a good source of well-absorbed **iron** and **zinc**, and **niacin**, and it also contains **potassium, phosphorus, riboflavin, vitamin B$_6$, vitamin B$_{12}$** and **folic acid**, as well as small amounts of **vitamin E**. See also **beefburger; mince; steak; stewing steak; hormones (in food)**.

beefburger A flat cake traditionally made of ground **beef** and seasonings, such as salt, pepper and herbs, and usually bound with flour and/or eggs. The nutritional and energy values of beefburgers vary according to their ingredients, and the cut of beef used to make them. In general they provide **protein**, **fat** with a high proportion of **saturated fatty acid** and most of the **micronutrients** associated with beef. Manufactured beefburgers are rarely made with 100% beef, but they must legally contain 52% lean meat, of which 80% must be beef. They may be given extra bulk by the addition of cereals, cereal fibre (bran) or soya fibre. They may also contain food additives. Few micronutrients are lost in frozen beefburgers, although there may be some losses of minerals **leached** out during thawing if they are not cooked direct from frozen. Beefburgers are usually fried or grilled. These cooking methods do not seriously deplete their nutritional content, but frying adds to their energy value.

beer An alcoholic drink usually made with malted barley, yeast and hops. The **alcohol** and **sugars** content and corresponding energy values of different beers vary. Low-alcohol beers, which contain less than 1% alcohol, are also available. See **ale**; **bitter**; **lager**; **shandy**; **stout**.

beet A group of related Eurasian plants, including a white-rooted variety used for the extraction of sugar (sugar beet), and a white-stemmed variety with green leaves eaten as a vegetable (spinach beet). Spinach beet provides **sugars**, **dietary fibre** and small amounts of **protein**. It also contains some **iron**, **manganese**, **carotene** and **folic acid**, and small amounts of **vitamin C**. See also **beetroot**.

beetroot The characteristically dark purple root of a variety of **beet** plant. Beetroot is eaten in salads, as a vegetable and as a pickle. It provides **sugars**, **dietary fibre** and some **protein**, **potassium**, and **folic acid**, and has an energy value of 44 kcal/ 100 g (boiled).

beriberi The characteristic deficiency disease of **thiamin**. It primarily affects the brain and nerves. Beriberi is prevalent in communities whose staple diet consists mainly of polished rice, but it is extremely rare in the UK, occurring among alcoholics. Its general symptoms are physical and mental weariness, loss of appetite and **oedema**, progressing to numbness and impaired sensations in the arms and legs. Walking becomes difficult as the muscles waste. Once the infection develops this far it is usually fatal, although in its early stages the disease is reversible and responds well to thiamin supplements.

bile A bitter, green-coloured alkaline solution containing **lecithin** and **cholesterol**. It is made in the liver, stored in the gall bladder and used in the duodenum (the first section of the intestines) to emulsify fats for digestion and absorption. Bile may be brought up during violent vomiting if the stomach is empty.

bioavailable A substance in a form that is readily utilized by the body's metabolic processes. The **nutrients** and **micronutrients** in foods are not always easily absorbed and assimilated (see **assimilation**) by the body, and some cooking or other processes may help make them more bioavailable, e.g. the nutrients and micronutrients in **pulses** are more bioavailable if the pulses are soaked to make sprouts. Although many cooking processes destroy vitamins, some cooking processes may make certain micronutrients more bioavailable, e.g. the **carotene** in cooked carrots is more bioavailable than in raw carrots.

biotin (also known as **vitamin H**) A **B complex vitamin**. Biotin is involved in the metabolism and energy release from nutrients. It is synthesized by intestinal bacteria in adults, and it is also obtained from the diet. It is found in offal, brown rice, nuts, fatty fish, brewer's yeast and egg yolks (raw egg whites contain a substance that prevents the absorption of biotin, and eggs should be cooked or separated to obtain the biotin content of the yolk). There is no UK **RDA**, but a daily intake of 150 to 200 μg is regarded as adequate. A biotin deficiency is rare because it is synthesized internally, but small children cannot synthesize it and may develop deficiencies typified by skin complaints, including **eczema**.

biscuit A small, flat, dry sweet or plain baked cake based on cereals but including a variety of different ingredients and flavourings. The nutritional and energy values of biscuits vary enormously according to their ingredients. Most biscuits are high in **starch** and **fat**, usually with a high proportion of **saturated fatty acids**. Sweet biscuits also contain **sugars** and all biscuits have high energy values. Manufactured biscuits may contain food additives.

bitter A **beer** with a characteristic bitter taste derived from its high hop content. Bitter contains between 3.0 and 3.6% alcohol by volume. It has an energy value of 32 kcal/100 g.

bitter lemon A sparkling lemon-flavoured soft drink. Bitter lemon is made with carbonated water, sugar and small amounts of lemon juice. It has an energy value of 35 kcal/100 ml and does not provide significant amounts of any **micronutrients**. It may contain artificial flavourings and colourings. **Low-calorie** bitter lemon is also available.

black treacle   A dark, viscous syrup obtained as a by-product of the crystallization of sugar, used as a spread or in desserts and cakes. It has a very high **sugar** content and a correspondingly high energy value of 257 kcal/100 g. It provides some **protein**, is rich in **potassium** and also contains some **calcium**, **magnesium**, **sulphur** and **chloride**.

blackberry   The fruit of the bramble made up of many tiny, soft, black, shiny-skinned pods on a small white core. Blackberries provide **dietary fibre**, **sugars**, small amounts of **protein** and have an energy value of 29 kcal/100 g. They are a good source of **vitamin C** and **E**, and also contain some **iron** and **carotene**. Some of the vitamin content is depleted if they are stewed, and, if they are stewed in sugar, their energy value is raised.

blackcurrant   The small fruit of a temperate shrub with thin, shiny black skin and juicy green flesh. Blackcurrants contain **dietary fibre**, **sugars**, small amounts of **protein** and have an energy value of 28 kcal/100 g. They are a good source of **vitamin C**, and they also provide **potassium**, **iron**, **carotene**, **biotin** and some **vitamin E**. The vitamin content is slightly depleted if they are stewed, and if they are stewed in sugar their energy value is raised.

blackcurrant drink A deep red cordial traditionally made with concentrated blackcurrant juice. Blackcurrant drink is a good source of **vitamin C**. It may contain added sugar and artificial flavourings and colourings. **Low-calorie** blackcurrant drinks are also available.

black pudding A mixture of pigs' blood, pork fat and cereals, stuffed into a pig's intestine and simmered. Similar in appearance to a sausage. It may be boiled, baked or fried before serving. Black pudding provides **protein**, a high **fat** content, with a high proportion of **saturated fatty acids**, and a high energy value at 305 kcal/100 g (fried). It is a very rich source of well-absorbed **iron** and a good source of **phosphorus**, **zinc**, **sulphur**, **biotin** and some **niacin**, **vitamin B$_{12}$** and **folic acid**. It has a very high **sodium** content.

blanching A method of pre-cooking food by immersing it in boiling water for a very short time. In the home, it may be used to help peel fruits (e.g. tomatoes) or nuts (e.g. almonds). It may be used to tenderize some vegetables (e.g. French beans, mangetout or courgettes) before using them in a salad or to remove unpleasant or strong tastes. Manufacturers blanch ingredients in the preparation of some canned foods and frozen foods. There is minimum loss of micronutrients as the process of blanching is so fast.

blood cell One of three different kinds of cells (red, white and platelet) made in the bone marrow and held in suspension in the blood plasma (the blood fluid). The red blood cells contain a complex iron compound called haemoglobin, which gives them their characteristic red colour. Haemoglobin transports oxygen from the lungs to the organs, muscles and other tissues. A number of dietary deficiencies can deplete the number of red blood cells, or cause malformation and impaired function, causing **anaemia**. There are fewer white blood cells, of which there are three different kinds. They all function as part of the immune system, destroying unwanted bacteria and preventing infection. Blood platelets are like granular fragments of red blood cells, and they are involved in the clotting of blood.

blood glucose The **glucose** in the blood. **Carbohydrates** in food are broken down to form glucose, which acts as a ready source of energy for all body tissues. The blood glucose level is monitored by hormones and is normally 0.8 to 1 g per litre. A rise in the level causes the pancreas to secrete **insulin**, which reduces the level by triggering the conversion of glucose to **glycogen**. If the blood glucose level drops below normal the pancreas secretes the hormone glucagon, which releases glucose from the glycogen stores in the liver. In situations of stress or danger the **adrenal gland** secretes adrenaline, which raises the blood glucose level in the same way. Low blood glucose levels cause fatigue, muscle weakness, and eventually unconsciousness and even coma. A sudden high intake of sugar can overstimulate the secretion of insulin and cause dramatic drops in blood glucose levels. The inability to secrete insulin (**diabetes**) causes very high blood sugar levels (hyperglycaemia) and excessive insulin activity causes very low blood sugar levels (hypoglycaemia).

blood pressure   The pressure that the flow of blood exerts on the artery walls. Blood pressure is affected by the force of the heart beat and the elasticity of the artery walls. **Hypertension** increases the risk of **heart disease** and stroke. Overweight and obese people are more likely to develop hypertension. A diet low in salt can be effective in reducing blood pressure in some people, but maintaining an acceptable body weight is the most effective.

body fat   The areas of **adipose tissue** in the body. Body fat is stored round organs such as the heart and kidneys to protect them, and under the skin as an energy store. It also acts as an insulator and so conserves body heat. Body fat accumulates if the energy requirements of the body are less than the energy supplied by the diet. For ways of reducing body fat, see APPENDIX I, LOSING AND GAINING WEIGHT.

body weight   The amount that a person weighs. Tables of acceptable body weight have been estab-

lished according to sex, height and body frame.
See APPENDIX I, LOSING AND GAINING WEIGHT, for a
table of acceptable body weight.

boiling A method of cooking, using boiling
water (100°C). Some vitamins are dstroyed by the
high temperature (e.g. **thiamin**, **vitamin C** and **pantothenic acid**), while others (e.g. **niacin**, **riboflavin**
and **vitamin B$_{12}$**) may be **leached** into the water.
Small amounts of mineral salts are also leached
into the water. To minimize these losses, food
should be boiled for only a short time in a minimum of water and, wherever possible, the cooking
water should be used in gravy or sauce. If the food
absorbs water during boiling (e.g. rice) the quantity of water should be calculated so that it is all
absorbed and none is discarded. Water drained
from boiling meat, fish or vegetables can be kept
and used as stock.

borage The young leaves of a Mediterranean
plant that are used in salads and as a herb. Borage
is usually used in such small quantities that its
nutritional properties are negligible, but the fresh
leaves, or an infusion of borage, are traditionally
used to alleviate fever by inducing perspiration.
The name borage is believed to be derived from
the Arabic words *abu araq*, 'father of sweat'.

bottle-feeding Feeding a baby from a bottle as
an alternative to breast-feeding. See APPENDIX II,
SPECIAL NEEDS.

brain The brain of a calf or lamb, eaten as **offal**. Brains provide **protein**, **fat** with a high proportion of **saturated fatty acids** and have an energy value of 110 kcal/100 g. They also contain **phosphorus**,. **iron**, **zinc**, **niacin**, **vitamin E**, **vitamin B₁₂**, **biotin**, and some **vitamin C**, **folic acid** and **pantothenic acid**. They have a high **sodium** level. Brains are usually fried, and this raises their energy value, causing some loss of the vitamin C and pantothenic acid.

braising A method of cooking in which the food, usually meat, is lightly fried and then allowed to simmer in a small amount of liquid in a closed container. It differs from stewing in that less water and larger cuts of meat are used. The frying, which enhances the flavour of the dish, may cause small losses of vitamins that are unstable at high temperatures, e.g. **thiamin** and **pantothenic acid**. However, the food is served in its juices and so the losses of micronutrients due to **leaching** are reduced.

bran The fibrous outer husk of cereals. The most common bran available is wheatbran, but bran can be taken from any cereal. Bran is very high in **dietary fibre** and most of it passes through the digestive system virtually unchanged, absorbing water and adding bulk to the faeces. It also contains **starch**, **protein**, a small amount of **fat** with a high proportion of **polyunsaturated fatty acids**, and an energy value of 206 kcal/100 g. It provides **potassium**, **phosphorus**, **niacin**, **folic acid**

and **biotin**, and some **copper**, **vitamin B₆** and **pantothenic acid**. Bran also contains **calcium**, **magnesium**, **iron** and **zinc**, but it also contains **phytic acid**, which inhibits the absorption of these minerals. It is preferable to consume bran naturally as part of the wholegrain rather than as a supplement. Phytic acid is destroyed in breadmaking and the wholegrain contains more minerals and vitamins than bran alone. It may be used in the treatment of constipation.

brandy A **spirit** made from distilled wine or champagne. Brandy contains 28 to 35% alcohol by volume. It has a fairly high **sugars** content and an energy value of 222 kcal/100 g.

brazil nut The crescent-shaped nut of a tropical South American tree with a woody, brown shell and an oily, off-white kernel. It has a high **fat** content with a high proportion of both **polyunsaturated** and **saturated fatty acids**. Brazil nuts provide **protein**, **dietary fibre**, some **sugars** and **starch**, and have an energy value of 619 kcal/100 g. They also contain **potassium**, **phosphorus**, **manganese**, small amounts of **copper** and most **B complex vitamins**. Brazil nuts contain **calcium**, **magnesium**, **iron** and **zinc**, but also **phytic acid**, which inhibits the absorption of these minerals.

bread A food made from a dough of flour which has been baked, usually after it has been raised. The energy value and nutritional properties of different kinds of bread vary because it can be prepared in different ways, and with many different ingredients. In general it is high in **starch**, and contains some **dietary fibre**, **sugars** and **protein**, and small amounts of **fat**. Wholemeal bread contains nearly three times as much dietary fibre as white bread and has an energy value of 216 kcal/100 g; white bread has an energy value of 233 kcal/100 g. Bread also contains **iron** and **zinc** and small amounts of most **B complex vitamins**. Most bread is made with salt and has a high **sodium** content.

The flour used is usually derived from wheat, but other cereals or mixed cereals may be used. White bread is made with refined flour, brown bread contains 85% wholegrain flour, wholemeal bread contains 100% wholegrain flour, and granary bread is similar to wholemeal bread, but it also contains whole grains of cereal. The higher the wholegrain content of the bread, the higher its dietary fibre, vitamin and mineral content. The flour is moistened to form a dough with water and/or milk, and the dough may also include eggs, sugar or malt extract. It may be raised using yeast or baking powder, or it may be unleavened, e.g. pitta bread. Many breads are permitted to contain food additives such as preservatives, raising agents and emulsifiers. Wholemeal bread is not permitted to contain additives except caramel for colour.

Bread may be sold as whole or sliced loaves or as buns, and it may or may not be packeted. When bread is toasted its energy value, weight for weight, is raised and there may be some small losses of vitamins that are unstable at high temperatures (e.g. **thiamin** and **pantothenic acid**).

breakfast cereal A general term for cereal products eaten with milk and possibly sugar, at breakfast time. The nutritional and energy values of breakfast cereals vary enormously according to the ingredients. They contain one or a mixture of several cereals. Some breakfast cereals are made with wholegrains, or contain added bran or wheatgerm, and have high **dietary fibre** contents, others are made with refined cereals and have lost much of their nutritional value. Breakfast cereals may be made with sugar or honey, and most of them contain salt. Some breakfast cereals also contain dried fruit or cocoa powder or other flavourings. Many breakfast cereals are fortified with vitamins and minerals, and they may contain food additives. Shoppers can check the ingredients and nutritional properties of breakfast cereals on the list of ingredients and the nutritional information given on the packet. See also **muesli**.

breast-feeding Feeding babies from the breast. When a woman is breast-feeding (lactating) her requirements for energy and some nutrients and micronutrients are increased. See APPENDIX II, SPECIAL NEEDS.

brewer's yeast The variety of yeast used in brewing beer. This by-product of the brewing process has a high **micronutrient** content and is sold as a food supplement in flake, powder or tablet form. It should not be confused with baker's yeast, which is live and would be harmful if eaten raw. The most widely available variety of brewer's yeast is torula yeast. It contains **protein**, minerals, trace elements and is a good source of **B complex vitamins**.

broad bean The ripe seed of a Eurasian bean plant, with a thin white skin and smooth green flesh. It is a **pulse** that is eaten as a vegetable. Broad beans provide **starch** and **dietary fibre**, some **protein** and small amounts of **sugars** and **fat**, and have an energy value of 48 kcal/100 g. They contain **potassium**, **manganese**, **carotene**, **pantothenic acid** and **biotin**, and some **iron**, **molybdenum** and **niacin**. Broad beans may contain small amounts of **phytic acid** and toxic **lectins**, and should be cooked thoroughly to destroy these harmful substances.

broccoli (also called **calabrese**) The green flower-head of a variety of cabbage that is eaten as a vegetable. Broccoli provides **dietary fibre**, **protein** and **sugars**, and has an energy value of 18 kcal/100 g (boiled). It is a good source of **calcium**, **potassium**, **carotene**, **vitamin C**, **riboflavin** and **folic acid**, and it also contains **iron**, **niacin**, **vitamin E**, **pantothenic acid**, **biotin** and **vitamin K**. The vitamin C and folic acid contents are depleted when it is boiled.

Brussels sprout The small, tight bud of a variety of cabbage eaten as a vegetable. Brussels sprouts provide **dietary fibre**, **sugars** and **protein**, and have an energy value of 18 kcal/100 g (boiled). They contain **potassium**, **carotene**, **vitamin C** and **folic acid**, and small amounts of **manganese**, **vitamin E** and **vitamin K**. The vitamin C and folic acid contents are depleted when they are boiled.

buckwheat The flour obtained from the seeds of the buckwheat plant. Buckwheat contains **starch**, some **protein** and **dietary fibre**, small amounts of **sugars** and **fat**, and has an energy value of 357 kcal/100 g. It is a good source of **molybdenum**, and also contains **potassium**, **iron**, **zinc**, **B complex vitamins** and **vitamin E**.

bulgar (also called **cracked wheat**) A form of wheat, in which the wholewheat grains are soaked and then roasted at very high temperatures until they crack. These pre-cooked grains need only a further 15–20 minutes to complete the cooking process. The nutritional content is similar to **wheat**.

bulimia nervosa A psychological disorder characterized by periods of compulsive eating, particularly of **carbohydrate** foods, followed by deliberate vomiting and/or laxative abuse to avoid gaining weight. Bulimia nervosa may have a number of psychological causes, and may develop in a person of either sex and at any age. It is most common among young women. Diarrhoea and vomiting **leach** the body of vitamins and minerals (particularly **potassium** and **magnesium**) and upset the body's **acid-base balance**. Sufferers are inclined to mood swings and to bouts of listlessness followed by hyperactivity. In women, the bizarre eating habits may cause menstruation to cease (amenorrhoea). Sufferers of bulimia nervosa must seek psychiatric treatment. See also **anorexia nervosa**.

butter A smooth, fatty, whitish-yellow paste obtained by churning cream from cows' milk and used for spreading on bread and for cooking. Butter is a concentrated form of **fat** and contains a high proportion of **saturated fatty acids**, and an energy value of 740 kcal/100 g. It is a good source of **vitamin A**, and also provides small amounts of high-quality **protein** and **vitamin D**. Butter may be plain, semi-salted or salted (which has a high **sodium** content).

butter bean The pale flat seed of a variety of bean of North American origin; a **pulse**. Butter beans provide **starch**, **dietary fibre**, **protein**, some **sugars**, small amounts of **fat** and have an energy value of 96 kcal/100 g (boiled). They also contain **potassium**, **iron**, **zinc** and small amounts of most **B complex vitamins**, but their vitamin content is lost when they are cooked. They may contain small amounts of **phytic acid** and **lectins**, and should be cooked thoroughly to destroy these harmful substances. Dried and canned butter beans have the same nutritional values as fresh ones, although canned beans may contain added salt and have a high **sodium** level.

buttermilk The sour watery liquid left when butter has been separated from cream, and sometimes used in cooking. Buttermilk has a high water content, but it provides some high-quality **protein**, **calcium**, **iron**, and **B complex vitamins**.

cabbage The large, leafy bud of certain varieties of a European plant. It has tightly packed, crisp white, green or purple leaves, or more loosely packed green leaves that may have a wrinkled texture. Cabbages are usually eaten boiled as vegetables, some (particularly white cabbage) are eaten raw in salads, and others (especially red cabbage) may be cooked in vinegar and spices. The nutritional values of most varieties of cabbage are similar. They have a high water content, provide only small amounts of **protein** and **sugars**, and have an energy value of approximately 23 kcal/100 g (raw) and 9 kcal/100 g (cooked). They are good sources of **potassium**, **vitamin C** and **folic acid**. Green cabbage also provides **carotene** and **calcium**. If cabbage is boiled, much of the potassium and folic acid are **leached** into the cooking water.

caffeine An organic substance naturally present in coffee, tea and the cola nut originally used in cola drinks. A daily intake of 250 mg caffeine (equivalent to 5 cups of tea or coffee) is usually sufficient to have a stimulant effect. At greater intakes it may accelerate the heart-rate, cause a jittery feeling in the muscles, lightheadedness and sleeplessness. Caffeine can be addictive and it can cause depression and irritability. It also has a **diuretic** effect.

calabrese See **broccoli**.

calcium The most abundant mineral in the body. It is found almost entirely in the bones and teeth, where it forms a hard structure. The calcium compounds in the bones are constantly being broken down and re-formed and the body requires a high dietary intake. The calcium in soft tissues controls the nerve impulses and muscle contractions. The UK **RDA** is 500 mg, and the requirement is higher for growing children and for pregnant and lactating women (see APPENDIX II, SPECIAL NEEDS). The best natural sources, of calcium are milk, cheese and yoghurt, sardines and white flour (which is fortified with calcium). Dark green vegetables are good sources, but some contain **oxalic acid**, which interferes with calcium absorption. The calcium in nuts and pulses is also not well absorbed because of the presence of **phytic acid**. Calcium stops accumulating in bones after about 35 years of age and to ensure the maximum amount of calcium in the bones at this stage, particular attention should be paid to calcium intakes up to this age. A large amount of calcium in the bones at middle-age helps to protect against the development of osteoporosis. Calcium deficiency caused by a low dietary intake, or a low vitamin D intake, causes **rickets** in children and **osteomalacia** in adults.

calorie A unit of heat, originally defined as the quantity of heat required to raise the temperature of 1 g of water by 1°C. The body's energy requirements and the energy value of food are measured in kilocalories (1000 calories) or kilojoules. If calorie is written with a capital C it is equivalent to a kilocalorie.

calorie counting A system of adding up the number of calories consumed on a daily basis. Calorie counting is a useful aid in a calorie-controlled diet for weight loss (or gain). See APPENDIX I, LOSING AND GAINING WEIGHT.

camomile tea A delicately flavoured, yellow infusion made with flowers from the camomile plant. Camomile tea is often used as an evening drink because it is believed to induce sleep and to aid digestion. It may also be used to bathe and soothe inflammations of the skin.

cancer A malignant growth or tumour caused by uncontrolled cell division. The exact causes of cancer are not known but diet is considered to be an important factor. A diet low in **saturated fats**

and high in **polyunsaturated fats** has been linked with reduced susceptibility to many forms of cancer (especially of the digestive system), as has a high intake of fruit, vegetables and wholegrain cereals. Cured foods and smoked foods may contain substances that can cause cancer. Smoking and alcohol are both known to increase susceptibility to cancer.

canned food Food that has been cooked and preserved in airtight cans. Nutrient losses are not great in this method of food preservation and only vitamin C is likely to be seriously depleted in canned foods. Salt and sugar are added to many canned foods, which increase the **sodium** levels and energy values. Many canned foods also contain a number of food additives.

capsicum Any of several varieties of tropical American plant with seeds used to make pepper. The seeds of a more spicy variety are used to make **cayenne pepper**, and the pod of a particularly pungent variety (**chilli peppers**) are used whole or ground to flavour foods. Some varieties have crisp red fruits that are eaten in salads or stuffed and cooked (see **peppers**).

caraway seed The long, thin, curved seed of a variety of Eurasian shrub. Caraway seeds are sprinkled over food, particularly bread, for their delicate flavour. They are eaten in such small quantities that their nutritional properties are negligible. They contain volatile oils which have traditionally been used to aid digestion and to act as an expectorant.

carbohydrate Any of a group of organic compounds, including **starch**, **polysaccharides** and **sugars**. They are important sources of energy for the body. The term 'complex carbohydrate' is applied to a carbohydrate containing both starch and **dietary fibre**. The carbohydrates are broken down into their component simple sugars during digestion: starches into **glucose**; **sucrose** into glucose and **fructose**; **lactose** into glucose and **galactose**. These simple sugars are either metabolized immediately to release energy, or stored as **glycogen** or body fat. All the various carbohydrates have a similar energy value of 4 kcal/1 g. It is recommended that for a healthy, balanced diet a greater amount of energy should be derived from starch and complex carbohydrates, rather than from sugars.

Foods rich in complex carbohydrates include wholegrain cereals and cereal products, fruit, vegetables and pulses. Foods rich in simple sugars include sucrose itself, honey, jam, confectionery, cakes and biscuits. See also the introductory chapter, A BALANCED DIET.

carnitine A substance synthesized in the liver and kidneys from the **amino acid** lysine, and also present in meat and dairy products. Carnitine is found in all parts of the body and exists in highest concentration in the muscles. It is essential to the transportation and oxidation of **fatty acids** within the body. If the body is deficient in **vitamin C**, carnitine synthesis may be seriously reduced; a deficiency can cause muscle weakness.

carob A cocoa substitute obtained from grinding the pod of a variety of evergreen Mediterranean tree. Carob tastes and looks similar to cocoa and is a little sweeter, but it contains none of the stimulants (**caffeine**, theophylline and a similar substance called theobromine) that are found in cocoa. Carob contains **sugars** and **starch**, and is rich in **calcium** and **potassium**. It has an energy value of 196 kcal/100 g.

carotene Any of a number of different substances (alpha-, beta- and gamma-carotene) that have the ability to be converted by the body into **retinol** (vitamin A). Carotene has a characteristically bright orange colour, and many good food sources are recognizable by this colour, e.g. carrots, cantaloup melon, apricots and pumpkin. Butter and dark green leafy vegetables are also good sources. There is no **RDA** for carotene but the dietary contribution and the poor absorption of carotene from foods that do not contain fat are taken into account in the RDA for vitamin A. There are no deficiency symptoms associated specifically with carotene as opposed to vitamin A. Excess intakes of carotene do not cause vitamin A toxicity, but they may cause yellowing of the skin, a condition that is reversible and harmless.

carrot The long, tapering orange root of a small shrub. Carrots may be eaten raw in salads, cooked as a vegetable or used in making moist cakes. They provide **sugars** and **dietary fibre**, and have an energy value of 19 kcal/100 g (boiled). They are a good source of **carotene** and also provide small amounts of **vitamin C** and **folic acid** (especially mature carrots). The carotene in carrots is more **bioavailable** if they are cooked, but cooking destroys some of the vitamin C content. Canned carrots contain less vitamin C and folic acid than fresh ones, and they may contain added salt and sugar.

cashew nut The fleshy, crescent-shaped nuts of a tropical American tree. Cashew nuts are not pleasant if eaten raw, and they are sold roasted. They have a high **fat** content, provide some **sugars**, **starch** and **dietary fibre**, and have an energy value of 571 kcal/100 g. They also contain **potassium**, **calcium**, **manganese**, **phosphorus**, **niacin** and **folic acid**, and a small amount of **iron**. Salted cashew nuts have a high **sodium** content.

cassava The starchy root of a tropical American plant. Cassava is cultivated for the extraction of **tapioca**. It is very high in **starch**, contains only small amounts of **protein** and micronutrients and has an energy value of 154 kcal/100 g (fresh).

cauliflower The tightly packed, fleshy white flower of a variety of cabbage. Cauliflower and its leaves are eaten boiled as a vegetable; the flower may also be eaten raw. Cauliflower has a high water content, provides small amounts of **protein**, **sugars** and **dietary fibre**, and has an energy value of 9 kcal/100 g (boiled). It also contains some **potassium**, **vitamin C** and **folic acid**. The leaves provide **manganese**, **calcium** and **carotene**. If cauliflower is boiled, about half of the potassium, vitamin C and folic acid are lost.

caviar The salted roe of sturgeon, a primitive bony fish of the northern hemisphere. There are many types of caviar (e.g. Beluga) obtained from different varieties of sturgeon. Their flavours vary, but their nutritional contents are virtually the same. Caviar provides **protein**, some **fat** and has an energy value of 268 kcal/100 g. It is a good source of **retinol**, and also contains **vitamin C**, **vitamin D**, **vitamin E** and some **vitamin B$_{12}$** and **biotin**. It is always highly salted, and has a very high **sodium** content.

cayenne pepper A particularly pungent, bright orange-red form of pepper, made from the ground seeds and pods of a variety of **capsicum**. It is eaten in such small quantities that its nutritional properties are negligible.

celeriac The hard, fibrous white root of a variety of celery. Celeriac is eaten raw in salads or boiled as a vegetable. It has a high water content, contains small amounts of **sugars**, **starch**, **dietary fibre** and **protein**, and has an energy value of 14 kcal/100 g (boiled). It also provides some **potassium** and small amounts of **iron** and **vitamin C**. About half the iron and vitamin C are lost when it is boiled. Celeriac may have a mild **diuretic** effect.

celery The crisp, fibrous white or green stalks of a Eurasian shrub. Celery is eaten raw in salads or boiled as a vegetable. It has a high water content, contains small amounts of **sugars**, **dietary fibre** and **protein**, and has an energy value of 8 kcal/100 g. It also provides **sodium**, **potassium** and **chloride**, and small amounts of **vitamin C** and **folic acid**. About half of all of these micronutrients is lost when celery is boiled.

cellulose A structural **polysaccharide** of **glucose**, found in the walls of plant cells. Cellulose gives the rigid structure to plants. It is a form of **dietary fibre** and is not broken down by digestive enzymes, although it may be partly fermented by intestinal bacteria.

cereal Any of a number of species of grass (e.g. wheat, oat, rice, maize, rye, barley and millet) that has an edible seed. Cereals are staple foods throughout the world. The term corn is used to mean the most common cereal in any particular country (in the UK corn, therefore, means wheat). Some cereals may be eaten whole, such as boiled rice, or young maize, and all of them can be ground to produce flour. However, only wheat and rye flour are suitable for making into bread because they contain sufficient **gluten**. Cereals are also used as a basis for breakfast cereals, e.g. cornflakes, puffed rice and porridge oats. Cereals are an important source of complex **carbohydrate**, most have a high **starch** content, and provide some **sugars** and **dietary fibre** (wholegrain cereals contain the highest levels). They also contain **protein, calcium, iron** and small amounts of most **B complex vitamins**. Wholegrain cereals are also rich in B complex vitamins and in addition contain **phosphorus, manganese** and **molybdenum**. Raw cereals may contain small amounts of **phytic acid**, and they should be cooked thoroughly in order to destroy this substance.

chapati   A flat, coarse unleavened bread usually eaten with Indian dishes. Chapatis are made with wheat flour. They provide **starch** and small amounts of **protein, sugars** and **dietary fibre**. They also contain some **calcium** and small amounts of **B complex vitamins**. Because they are made with dough that has not risen, they may contain some **phytic acid**.

cheese   The curd of milk separated from the whey and treated with rennet and often salt, allowed to clot and sometimes to mature and ferment, to produce a pasty, tangy substance. Rennet is a substance made from the enzyme rennin (derived from calves' stomach), a vegetable rennet (derived from plants) is also available. There are an enormous variety of cheeses; France alone has a different cheese for every day of the year. The variations are obtained by using different milk (usually cows' milk but also goats' and ewes' milk), by introducing different bacteria or moulds at the fermentation stage, and by leaving the paste to develop for a specific length of time. The general types of cheese are, hard, soft, crumbly and elastic. They may include other ingredients, such as herbs or chopped nuts. The blue areas in some blue cheeses are made by moulds, in others they are achieved by introducing copper wires into the maturing paste.

All cheeses provide a good source of **protein**. The **fat** content, which has a high proportion of **saturated fatty acids**, and the energy value of cheeses varies enormously. Cottage cheese has a very low fat content and an energy value of 96 kcal/100 g, and Stilton a very high fat content and an energy value of 462 kcal/100 g. In general cheese has a fairly high energy value, and in hard cheeses it tends to be higher than in soft varieties (some cheeses are labelled 'full fat', 'medium fat' or 'low fat'). Reduced fat cheeses are available for many of the common types of cheese. Most cheeses are rich in **calcium**, **vitamin A** and **riboflavin**. Cheeses made from vegetable oils and from soya milk are also available and are particularly suitable for **vegans**. See also **curd cheese**.

cherry A small rounded fruit with bright red or deep purple skin, sweet, juicy reddish flesh and a small hard stone. Most cherries are eaten fresh, some less sweet varieties are stewed or used in pies, and they may be crystallized in sugar (glacé cherries) or used to give flavour and as a garnish to desserts and cakes. Cherries provide **sugars**, small amounts of **dietary fibre** and have an energy value of 47 kcal/100 g. They also contain **potassium**, **vitamin A**, **folic acid** and **vitamin C**. Stewed, canned and glacé cherries contain much less **folic acid** and vitamin C. Glacé cherries contain a lot of sugar and have a higher energy value. Maraschino cherries are preserved in a liqueur made from the cherries themselves and provide very little of the vitamin content of fresh cherries.

chervil The leaves of a small Eurasian shrub that have a pleasant aniseed flavour and are used fresh in salads or dried and used as a herb. Chervil is eaten in such small quantities that its nutritional properties are negligible.

chestnut The nut of a variety of chestnut tree (sweet chestnut) that has a smooth, tough brown skin and wrinkled-looking yellowish flesh. Raw chestnuts are not edible, and they are usually roasted or boiled. They may be crystallized in sugar (marron glacés) and eaten as a delicacy. Chestnuts provide **starch**, **sugars**, **dietary fibre**, small amounts of **protein** and contain less **fat** than other nuts, and have a comparatively low energy value of 170 kcal/100 g. They also contain **potassium**, **manganese** and a small amount of **biotin**. None of these micronutrients is seriously depleted if they are baked, boiled or glacéed. Marrons glacés contain a lot of sugar and have a high energy value.

chicken A domestic fowl and its meat. It provides **protein** and little **fat** (white meat has a lower proportion of **saturated fatty acid** than red meat). The fat is mainly in the skin, and the fat content and energy value can be reduced if the skin is removed before or after cooking. Chicken also provides **potassium**, **phosphorus**, **sulphur**, **niacin** and **folic acid**, and some **zinc**, **pantothenic acid** and **biotin** (the dark meat contains more than the breast). None of these micronutrients are seriously depleted when chicken is cooked.

chickpea The small, whitish pea-shaped seed of a leguminous plant grown mostly in Mediterranean countries and central Asia; it is a **pulse**. Chickpeas are usually boiled and eaten whole or boiled, pulped and spiced to make **dahl** or ground to make **hummus**. They contain **starch**, **protein**, **dietary fibre** and **sugars**, and have an energy value of 142 kcal/100 g (boiled). They also provide **potassium**, **calcium**, **magnesium**, **manganese**, **carotene** and **folic acid** and small amounts of **fat**, **iron** and **niacin**. Some of the carotene and folic acid is lost when chickpeas are cooked or canned. If canned chickpeas contain added salt they have a high **sodium** content.

chickweed A small, common, white-flowered garden weed with small rounded leaves that is sometimes eaten boiled as a vegetable. Chickweed has a high water content and provides only small amounts of **sugars**, **dietary fibre** and **protein**. It is rich in **potassium** and also provides some **iron** and **carotene**.

chicory The tightly packed bud of a small blue-flowered plant, with yellow-green leaves on wide, crisp white stems. Chicory leaves are eaten in salads, or boiled and eaten as a vegetable. The leaves have a very high water content, provide small amounts of **protein** and **dietary fibre**, and have an energy value of 9 kcal/100 g. They also contain **folic acid** and a small amount of **vitamin C**. Much of the vitamin content is lost when they are cooked. Chicory root is ground and used as a cheap, caffeine-free coffee substitute.

chilli peppers The red or green and red tapering pod of a particularly pungent variety of **capsicum**, used whole or ground to flavour foods. Chillies are eaten in such small quantities that their nutritional values are negligible.

China tea Any variety of **tea** of Chinese origin. China tea is usually more delicate and fragrant than Indian or Kenyan tea, but it contains the same amount of **caffeine** and theophylline. It is rich in manganese.

Chinese leaf A variety of cabbage with a tall tightly packed bud of wrinkled pale green leaves on crisp, wide white stems. Chinese leaf is usually eaten in salads, but it may be boiled and eaten as a vegetable. It has a very high water content, provides negligible amounts of **sugars**, **dietary fibre** and **protein**, and has an energy value of 25 kcal/100 g. It also contains small amounts of **folic acid** and **vitamin** C. Much of the vitamin content is lost if it is boiled.

Chinese restaurant syndrome A condition, developed by some people, usually attributed to the large quantities of **monosodium glutamate** used in Chinese cooking. Its symptoms include a burning sensation across the back of the neck, tightness in the chest, sweating and headaches. In most cases, the symptoms are not serious and do not last more than a few hours.

chip A strip of potato that is traditionally cooked by deep-frying. Chips have a very high **fat** content as they absorb fat during frying and a correspondingly high energy value of 253 kcal/100 g. They provide most of the nutrients and micronutrients associated with **potatoes** (starch, protein, dietary fibre, potassium, niacin and vitamin B_6). 'Oven-ready' chips, which are pre-prepared and cooked by baking, usually have a lower fat content and energy value.

chive The thin tubular leaves of a small, purple-flowered Eurasian plant. Chives have a mild onion flavour, and are chopped and used fresh or dried to give flavour to foods. They are consumed in very small quantities and their nutritional values are negligible.

chlorella A variety of green alga. Chlorella contains **protein**, **sugars** and some **fat**, as well as **iron**, **iodine**, **zinc**, **cobalt**, **carotene** and **vitamin B₁₂**. It also contains a high percentage of cholorophyll, the green pigment in plants that enables them to use the energy in sunlight to synthesize carbohydrates. Chlorella may be used as a dietary supplement, although its beneficial properties are not universally acknowledged.

chloride A non-metallic mineral essential to humans. With **sodium**, chloride is involved in maintaining the water balance in the body. It combines with hydrogen to form hydrochloric acid, which is found in the digestive juices in the stomach. There is no UK **RDA** for chloride, but nutritionists in the United States estimate that a daily intake of 1700–5000 mg is adequate. The primary source of chloride intake is common **salt**, either added during cooking, processing or at the table, or in salty foods (e.g. cheese, canned foods, meat products, cured meats, smoked foods, fish, bread, biscuits, pastries and breakfast cereals). Chloride deficiency only occurs where there is a correspondingly low sodium intake, unless there is some other underlying illness or disease. Chloride is excreted in the urine and there is no danger of toxic levels accumulating in the body.

chocolate A hard, dark-brown paste made from ground cocoa seeds that have been roasted and sweetened with sugar. Milk chocolate also contains dried or condensed milk, and chocolate may contain natural or artificial flavourings. Chocolate is eaten by itself or combined with biscuits, dried fruits and/or nuts, and it is used in many cakes and desserts. It has a high sugar and fat content, with a high proportion of **saturated fatty acids**, and a correspondingly high energy value of 529 kcal/100 g (milk chocolate). It has a high **sodium** content, and provides some **potassium**, **calcium** (more in milk chocolate), **iron** (more in plain chocolate) and **folic acid**. It also contains small amounts of theobromine (a substance very similar to caffeine that acts as a stimulant).

cholecalciferol (also called **vitamin D₃**) The form of **vitamin D** produced by the action of ultra-violet rays in sunlight on **cholesterol** in the skin .

cholesterol A fatty substance that occurs naturally in all animal tissues, including the bloodstream. Most of the cholesterol is made in the liver from **saturated fatty acids**. Smaller amounts are obtained from the diet, particularly from eggs, liver, kidney and roe. Cholesterol is an important constituent of cell membranes and the fatty sheath that protects the nerves, and is also used by the body in the synthesis of **bile** and of hormones. Cholesterol is carried in the blood as **lipoproteins**. High levels of low-density lipoproteins (LDL) are associated with an increased risk of **coronary heart disease**. Eating less fat, particularly fat with a high proportion of saturated fatty acids can help to lower the LDL levels. To a lesser extent, increasing the intake of fats with a high proportion of **polyunsaturated fatty acids** can also assist in reducing the level. See the introductory chapter, A BALANCED DIET.

choline Part of the phospholipid **lecithin**, and incorrectly classed as part of the **B complex vitamins**. Choline is made in the body and although found in large quantities in food (especially liver, egg yolk and wheatgerm) it is not an essential nutrient.

chop A cut of meat from the loin of mutton, lamb or pork, usually including a rib or vertebra. The nutritional and energy values of chops vary according to the animal, and to the part of the spine from which they are taken. In general they contain **protein** and **fat**, with a high proportion of **saturated fatty acids**. The fat content of chops can be reduced by trimming away visible fat before or after cooking. They usually also provide **phosphorus**, well-absorbed **zinc** and **iron**, **niacin**, **riboflavin**, **thiamin** and **vitamin B$_{12}$**. Chops may be grilled, roasted or fried. Grilled chops have a lower fat content and energy value than roasted or fried ones. Some niacin, riboflavin and thiamin may be **leached** into the fat while chops are cooking.

chromium A metallic **trace element** essential to humans. Chromium is necessary for the metabolism of **glucose** because it helps activate **insulin**, and is part of a substance called Glucose Tolerance Factor (GTF), which is synthesized by the body. Chromium supplements are, therefore, used in the treatment of some forms of **diabetes**. It is also involved in the metabolism and transportation of **fats**. There is no **RDA** for chromium, but in the United States a daily intake of 50–200 μg is considered adequate.

Chromium is found in shellfish, fish, meat, molasses, rice bran, egg yolk and brewer's yeast. The use of stainless steel cooking containers and implements, which contain chromium, may contribute to the intake in the diet. Refined and processed foods contain much lower levels of chromium than fresh products. Chromium deficiency is rare because it is needed in such small quantities. However, a diet high in refined and processed foods could cause a deficiency typified by nervousness and susceptibility to diabetes, and raised blood **cholesterol** levels. Excess chromium intake is also rare, but it could be caused by overuse of chromium supplements. An excess, as with other minerals, is toxic and causes nausea vomiting and diarrhoea.

chutney A type of **pickle**, originally from India, made with ripe or unripe fruit, vinegar, sugar, salt and spices. The nutritional properties and energy values of chutneys vary according to their ingredients. In general, they provide **sugars** and small amounts of **dietary fibre**. They have fairly high energy values because of the sugar content, and they may provide small amounts of the micronutrients associated with the fruit used. Chutneys are acidic because of the vinegar content, and they usually contain salt and, therefore, have a high **sodium** content. Manufactured chutneys may contain food **additives**, especially colourings and flavourings.

cider Fermented apple juice that is allowed to mature for specific periods of time so that more, or less, of the **sugars** turn to alcohol. Cider contains alcohol (about 4% by volume in dry cider and 3.7% by volume in sweet varieties) and sugars (more in sweet than dry varieties). It does not contain significant amounts of any micronutrients. Dry cider has an energy value of 36 kcal/100 g. Vintage cider has a much higher alcohol content (more than 10% by volume) and a higher sugars content. It has a correspondingly higher energy value of 101 kcal/100 g.

cider vinegar The mild, pleasantly flavoured vinegar obtained as a by-product of cider. Cider vinegar is milder than other vinegars because it only contains about 5% by volume of **acetic acid**. It also contains traces of minerals. Cider vinegar is traditionally used as an astringent for cleansing and stimulating the digestive system.

cinnamon The fragrant, yellow-brown bark of a

tropical Asian tree that is ground and used as a spice. Cinnamon is used in such small quantities that its nutritional properties are negligible. Cinnamon infusions have a pleasant, delicate flavour, and have traditionally been used as a mild disinfectant and stimulant.

cirrhosis A degenerative disease that affects the organs, most commonly the liver, causing the cells of the organ to harden and die until large portions of the organ can no longer function. Cirrhosis may be caused by bacterial or viral infections or inadequate diet, but in the UK it is more commonly caused by excessive alcohol consumption. The liver has a great capacity to recover, but if cirrhosis is not treated and the cause of the disease not isolated and eliminated, it can eventually be fatal.

citric acid A mild acid found in many fruits, especially citrus fruits. Citric acid is involved in the metabolism of foods to release energy. It is also used as a food additive in jams and soft drinks to give a tart flavour.

citrus fruit The fruits of certain varieties of tropical and subtropical trees and shrubs, characterized by a waxy yellow or orange rind and mildly acid, juicy flesh in crescent-shaped segments. Citrus fruits have a higher **citric acid** content than other fruits, and most of them are good sources of **vitamin C**. See **clementine**; **grapefruit**; **lemon**; **lime**;

mandarin; orange; satsuma; tangerine; ugli fruit.

clementine A small citrus fruit with shiny orange skin and sweet, juicy orange flesh in crescent-shaped segments with many small pips. The clementine was originally obtained by crossing a tangerine with a sweet variety of orange. Clementines provide **sugars** and **dietary fibre**, and have an energy value of 46 kcal/100 g. They contain **vitamin C** and smaller amounts of **vitamin B₆ and folic acid**. All of these micronutrients are seriously depleted if clementines are canned.

clove A pungent, immature flower bud of a tropical evergreen tree that is dried and used whole or ground as a spice. Cloves are consumed in such small quantities that their nutritional properties are negligible.

cob nut A variety of **hazelnut**.

cobalamin See **vitamin B₁₂**.

cobalt A metallic element that is an important constituent of **vitamin B₁₂**. Cattle and sheep have intestinal bacteria that can synthesize **vitamin B₁₂** using cobalt, but it cannot be synthesized in the human body and the vitamin must be obtained from food sources. In humans, there are no known functions for cobalt other than in **vitamin B₁₂** and there is no **RDA** for cobalt or any deficiency symptoms specific to it. Levels of cobalt in food are too low to constitute any danger of toxicity, but food additives containing cobalt have been banned because toxic levels of this metal can be fatal.

cockle   A mollusc shellfish with a rounded shell, usually eaten boiled. Cockles provide **protein**, very little **fat** and have an energy value of 50 kcal/100 g (boiled). They also contain **calcium**, **phosphorus**, **iron** and **zinc**. They are usually boiled in sea water or highly salted water, and have a very high **sodium** content.

cocoa powder   A fine, dark brown powder obtained by roasting and grinding husked cocoa beans, the seeds of the cacao tree. Cocoa powder is used to make hot drinks and for flavouring biscuits, cakes and desserts. It provides **protein**, **fat** with a high proportion of **saturated fatty acids** and has an energy value of 312 kcal/100 g. It is rich in **calcium** and **potassium**, and has a high **sodium** content. Cocoa also contains **caffeine** and theobromine (a stimulant related to caffeine).

coconut   The large, hard stone of the green fibrous fruit of the coconut palm, with a ropy, woody shell lined with a kernel of crisp, white, delicately flavoured flesh and clear yellowish fluid. Coconuts are used commercially for the extraction of coconut oil. The flesh can be eaten fresh or dried, and desiccated coconut is used for flavouring food. Coconut flesh has a high **saturated fatty**

acid content, provides **dietary fibre** and small amounts of **protein** and **sugars**, and has an energy value of 351 kcal/100 g. It also contains **potassium** and **folic acid**. All of the folic acid is lost in desiccated coconut, which has a higher energy value of 604 kcal/100 g. Coconut milk contains some sugars but has virtually no micronutrient content.

coconut oil A vegetable oil obtained from the flesh of coconuts. Coconut oil contains a high proportion of **saturated fatty acids**, and is used in the manufacture of soaps and cosmetics as well as in commercial cooking processes. Like all oils, it is almost pure fat and has an energy value of 899 kcal/100 g.

cod A white fish from the North Atlantic, usually sold as fillets or steaks. Cod can be served in a variety of ways: baked, grilled, poached, steamed, fried or deep fried in batter. Cod provides **protein**, very little **fat** and has an energy value of 80 kcal/100 g (steamed). It also provides well-absorbed **iron** and **zinc**, **potassium**, **phosphorus**, **sulphur**, vitamin B_{12}, **folic acid**, **biotin** and some **niacin**. When cod is fried or deep fried, it has a higher energy value of 199 kcal/100 g and the sulphur and all of the vitamins are lost. The micronutrient contents are not seriously affected by any other cooking methods.

cod-liver oil The oil extracted from the liver of cod and related fish. Cod-liver oil is a rich source of **vitamin A** and **vitamin D**, and is used, particularly for children, as a supplement. It is high in unsaturated **fatty acids** and contains some **polyunsaturated fatty acids**. It has a high energy value of 800 kcal/100 ml.

coeliac disease An intestinal disorder (possibly hereditary) caused by an intolerance to **gluten** (found principally in wheat, but also in rye). Some coeliac patients are also unable to tolerate barley and oats. Coeliac disease most commonly affects children but it can be diagnosed at any age. The presence of gluten in the diet causes the development of lesions in the small intestine resulting in poor absorption of fats, which causes foul-smelling, fatty diarrhoea. The lesions may also interfere with the absorption of iron, **vitamin B₁₂, vitamin D** and **vitamin K**, causing deficiencies of these micronutrients. Untreated the symptoms are poor growth and **rickets** in children, weight loss and **osteomalacia** in adults, and **anaemia**. Treatment involves removing wheat and rye from the diet, and in some cases also barley and oats, or any products made from these cereals.

coffee A hot drink made by infusing the roasted, ground seeds ('beans') of the coffee tree. Coffee can be bought as whole roasted beans, ready-ground beans or 'instant' coffee (where the infusion has been made and freeze-dried to form granules or powder). It may be drunk black or with milk, and with or without sugar. Black unsweetened coffee has no energy value. It provides some **potassium**, **magnesium** and small amounts of **niacin**. It also contains the stimulant **caffeine** (about 125 mg in the average cup of fresh coffee, or 70 mg in instant coffee). Decaffeinated coffee is also available. It is not caffeine-free but contains only about 4 mg of caffeine per average cup.

cola drink A sweet, dark brown, carbonated (fizzy) drink traditionally flavoured with cola nuts (the seeds of a tropical tree). Cola drinks provide **sugars**, have a high energy value of 39 kcal/100 g, but do not contain significant amounts of any micronutrients. Most cola drinks contain **caffeine**. Low-calorie cola drinks, with artificial **sweeteners** and caffeine-free, are also available.

coley See **saithe**.

comfrey tea An infusion of the leaves of a small Eurasian plant. Comfrey tea is mildly astringent and has traditionally been used to stop diarrhoea, and in the treatment of ulcers.

common salt See **salt**.

confectionery Any of numerous kinds of sweet foods, made wholly or partly from sugar. Many forms of confectionery, e.g. boiled sweets, are made with crystallized boiled sugar with added flavouring and colourings. Because sugar is the main ingredient of most forms of confectionery, they have energy values similar to sugar of 112 kcal/100 g and virtually no **micronutrient** content. Reduced calorie confectionery is virtually impossible to make because most sweets rely on sugar for their bulk and structure as well as for the characteristic sweetness. Sweets may also contain other ingredients such as fruit juice, pieces of fruit or nut, liquorice, aniseed, chocolate and condensed milk. Many kinds of sweet contain **artificial colouring** and **flavourings**.

conserve   See **jam**.

consommé   A clear soup made from **stock** of meat, poultry, game or fish. The nutritional properties of consommé vary according to the stock it is made from, but in general it provides some **protein** and very little **fat**, and has a correspondingly low energy value. It may also contain small amounts of micronutrients **leached** into the stock. Consommé is usually highly salted and therefore has a high **sodium** content. Canned consommé may contain colouring and flavourings.

constipation   Infrequent, difficult and sometimes painful evacuation of the bowels, with hard faeces. Constipation is usually caused by a lack of **dietary fibre** in the diet. Some dietary fibre, particularly from wholegrain cereals, absorbs water as it passes undigested down the digestive tract and adds bulk and moisture to the stools, encouraging regular and comfortable evacuation of the bowels. Occasional, acute constipation can be treated with **laxatives**. If the symptoms are permanent and do not improve with an increased intake of dietary fibre, medical advice should be sought.

convenience food   Food that needs little preparation and can be used at any time. Many convenience foods are pre-cooked and canned, chilled or frozen. They can be served straight from the packaging, or need only re-heating. It is important to follow the manufacturer's cooking instructions carefully. The nutritional and energy values of convenience foods vary according to their ingredients and the degree of processing. They may also contain food **additives**.

cooking   The preparing of food by heating it. There are many different methods of cooking, and many of them alter the nutritional value of foods, e.g. cooking with oil adds to the energy value of foods because they absorb oil, and cooking at high temperatures destroys some vitamins that are unstable to heat. See **baking**; **barbecuing**; **blanching**; **boiling**; **braising**; **deep frying**; **frying**; **grilling**; **leaching**; **parboil**; **roasting**.

cooking fat   Any form of **fat** that is suitable for cooking, e.g. dripping, lard and suet. Cooking fat is solid at room temperature and this indicates that it is high in **saturated fatty acids**. Fats with a high proportion of unsaturated fatty acids and

polyunsaturated fatty acids, e.g. polyunsaturated margarine and oil, may be used in cooking as a healthier alternative. Cooking fats have a very high energy value of approximately 890 kcal/100 g.

cooking oil Any kind of oil that is suitable for cooking, e.g. sunflower oil and groundnut oil. Cooking oil, which is usually made of vegetable oils, is liquid at room temperature, and most are high in **polyunsaturated fat**.

copper An essential, metallic **trace element**, found mostly in the liver, kidneys and brain. Copper encourages the absorption of **iron** and the formation of red blood cells. It is also an important constituent of a number of **enzymes**. There is no **RDA** for copper, but it is generally accepted that a daily intake of 2–3 mg is adequate. The best sources are shellfish, liver, some nuts, olives, pulses, wholegrain cereals and brewer's yeast. Copper may also be obtained from soft water that has passed through copper pipes, or foods that have been processed or stored in copper containers. Copper deficiencies are rare, but they may be caused by a diet high in processed foods, or they may arise after continued diarrhoea. The symptoms of a deficiency include **anaemia**, **oedema**, loss of hair colour and condition, and increased susceptibility to bone fractures. The danger of toxicity is also rare, but it can occur in Wilson's disease (a hereditary disease) and is characterized by diarrhoea, vomiting, pain in the abdomen and poor kidney function.

cordial (also called **squash**) A refreshing drink made with fruit juice or fruit syrup diluted with water. Cordials are traditionally made with concentrated fruit juice and sugar. Many manufactured cordials contain very little true fruit juice, but they do contain sugar, and have a correspondingly high energy value of approximately 112 kcal/100 g (undiluted). **Low-calorie** cordials are also available. They may contain colouring and flavourings, and some may also contain added vitamins, e.g. some forms of blackcurrant drink are enriched with **vitamin C**.

coriander The dried ripe seeds of a Eurasian shrub that are used to give flavour to food; the leaves may also be used. Coriander is used in such small quantities that its nutritional properties are negligible.

corn A name given to the kind of cereal that is most commonly found in any particular country. In the UK corn usually means wheat, or it may refer to maize, e.g. corn on the cob.

corn oil The yellow-coloured vegetable oil extracted from maize and used for cooking. It has a high **polyunsaturated fatty acids** content, including a high percentage of **linoleic acid**, an energy value of 899 kcal/100 g and contains **vitamin E**.

corn on the cob See **sweetcorn**.

cornflour A fine, starchy flour made from maize and used for thickening foods, especially sauces. Cornflour has a very high **starch** content, an energy value of 354 kcal/100 g and provides no other nutrients or micronutrients.

coronary heart disease A general name for a number of heart conditions usually caused by **atherosclerosis** of the coronary artery, which supplies blood and oxygen to the muscles of the heart. Coronary heart disease may include the degeneration and death of part of the heart muscle tissue, and may cause angina (acute pain in the chest and breathlessness). In serious cases, it can lead to cardiac arrest and can be fatal. Susceptibility to coronary heart disease is higher in the elderly, in the obese, in those who take little exercise and those who suffer from diabetes. Men are more susceptible to it than pre-menopausal women. The likelihood of developing coronary heart disease is increased if blood **cholesterol** levels are high, or if a person has **hypertension** or smokes. To minimize the risks, total **fat** intake should be reduced, particularly those fats with a high proportion of **saturated fatty acids**, and the fat that is eaten should have a high proportion of **polyunsaturated fatty acids**. Also regular exercise should be taken, and smoking should be avoided.

cottage cheese A mild-tasting, soft white cheese with a loose, lumpy texture, made from skimmed milk. Cottage cheese provides **protein**, small amounts of **sugars**, and is valued for its very low **fat** content and correspondingly low energy value of 96 kcal/100 g. Some cottage cheese is made with added cream and contains about 4% fat by weight, otherwise it contains just 0.4% by weight. It contains some **phosphorus**, **retinol**, **carotene**, **niacin** and **folic acid**. Like most cheeses, cottage cheese is usually made with salt and has a high **sodium** content.

courgette A small variety of marrow with thin, shiny, dark green skin and pithy whitish flesh. Courgettes can be eaten raw in salads, but they are usually boiled or fried and eaten as vegetables. They have a high water content, provide only small amounts of **sugars**, **dietary fibre**, **starch** and **protein**, and have an energy value of 25 kcal/100 g. They also contain some **potassium**, **carotene**, **vitamin C** and **folic acid**. Most of the potassium and folic acid and some of the vitamin C are lost if they are boiled, and virtually all of these micronutrients are lost if they are fried.

couscous Fine or coarse grains of millet, steamed and eaten with meat dishes to give bulk to meals, or used as a basis for salads. Couscous is high in **starch** and **sugars**, provides some **protein** and has an energy value of 227 kcal/100 g. It also contains some **sulphur**, **chloride** and **folic acid**. Some of the folic acid content is lost when it is steamed.

75

crab A marine crustacean shellfish, usually pink or brown, with a broad, flat shell, pincers and smooth, tangy flesh. Crab is usually steamed or boiled and served chilled with salad or hot with a sauce. It provides **protein**, some **fat** and has an energy value of 127 kcal/100 g. It also contains **potassium, phosphorus, iron, copper, zinc, sulphur, chloride, folic acid, pantothenic acid** and **niacin**. It has a high **sodium** content. Some of the vitamin content is lost when it is cooked. Canned crab contains less fat, potassium, phosphorus, copper and niacin than fresh crab, and none of the sulphur, folic acid or pantothenic acid. It contains more calcium and iron, and has a higher sodium content.

crab stick See **seafood stick**.

cranberry The sour red berry of a variety of trailing shrub. Cranberries are usually too sour to eat fresh, but they are made into jam or jelly and are sometimes served with meat, especially turkey. They provide **sugars, dietary fibre**, small amounts of **protein** and have an energy value of 15 kcal/100 g. They are a good source of **iron**, and contain some **vitamin C** and **folic acid**. Most of the vitamin C and folic acid contents are lost when they are cooked or made into jams and jellies.

cream The yellow fat that rises to the top of milk if it is allowed to stand and which is removed when milk is skimmed. Cream is used in cooking and for adding to desserts. It has a high **fat** content, with a high proportion of **saturated fatty acid**, and has a correspondingly high energy value. There are different kinds of cream with varying fat contents: clotted cream with the highest fat content of more than 50% by weight and an energy value of 593 kcal/100 g; double cream with 48.2% and an energy value of 447 kcal/100 g; whipping cream with 35% and single cream with 21.2%, both with an energy value of 212 kcal/100 g. Cream also provides small amounts of **sugars** and **protein**. It is rich in **vitamin A** (more in clotted, less in single) and contains some **potassium**, **calcium**, **folic acid** and **biotin**.

cream cheese A smooth, soft white cheese made from cream or whole milk and used in cooking. The fat content, nutritional and energy value of cream cheese depend on the fat content of the milk or cream it was made from. Shoppers should check the labels, which usually indicate what percentage of cream cheese is fat.

crème fraiche Cream that has been allowed to sour slightly and to acquire a cheesy tang. Crème fraiche is available with different fat contents, and shoppers should check labels, which usually indicate what percentage of crème fraiche is fat.

crispbread A thin dry, unsweetened biscuit made of wheat or rye. There are many different kinds of crispbreads, but in general they provide

starch, **dietary fibre**, some **protein**, **sugars** and **fat**.
They also contain **potassium**, **phosphorus**, **iron**,
zinc, **niacin** and **folic acid**. They are valued by slimmers for their low energy value. Starch-reduced
crispbreads are also available, and these have a
lower energy value. Crispbreads with a high dietary fibre content are also available. Most crispbreads are made with salt and have high **sodium**
contents.

crisp A very thin slice of potato, fried and eaten
cold as a snack, or traditionally served hot with
game. Crisps are high in **starch** and **fat**, and have a
correspondingly high energy value of 533 kcal/100
g (thicker cut crisps have a lower fat content, and
energy value – weight for weight – than other
crisps). Crisps also provide **dietary fibre** and **protein** and are rich in **potassium**, and contain some
iron, **niacin**, **vitamin C**, **vitamin E** and **folic acid**.
They are usually highly salted and have a very
high **sodium** content. They may be flavoured with
vinegar or with other flavourings and contain
other food additives. Low-fat and low-salt crisps
are also available, as are crisps in which the potato
skin has been retained (these are higher in dietary
fibre).

cucumber The long, thin fruit of a creeping
plant, with thin, smooth or ridged, dark green
skin and juicy, translucent, greenish flesh. Cucumber is eaten raw in salads, and small or immature
cucumbers are sometimes pickled (see **gherkins**).

It has a very high water content, provides only very small amounts of **sugars** and **protein**. and has an energy value of 10 kcal/100 g. It also contains **folic acid** and some **potassium** and **vitamin C**.

cumin The aromatic seeds of a Mediterranean shrub, dried and used whole or ground to give flavour to food. Cumin is used in such small quantities that its nutritional properties are negligible.

curd cheese A smooth, mild-tasting white cheese made from skimmed or semi-skimmed milk. Curd cheese is used in cooking, and, unlike **cottage cheese**, it is stirred during the brief maturing period to give it its smooth texture. The **fat** content of curd cheese is usually higher than cottage cheese, but it varies and shoppers should check labels, which usually indicate what percentage of curd cheese is fat.

curing A method of preserving meat, fish and game by salting and/or smoking (see **smoked foods**). Cured foods usually retain most of the nutrients and micronutrients of the equivalent fresh food. Although, if curing has involved smoking there may some losses of vitamins that are unstable at high temperatures, e.g. **thiamin** and **pantothenic acid**. Cured foods are highly salted and have very high **sodium** contents. They usually contain **nitrates** and **nitrites** and colouring and flavourings.

currant A dried blackcurrant used in biscuits and cakes. Currants have a high **sugars** content (mostly as glucose and fructose) provide some **dietary fibre** and **protein**, and have an energy value of 243 kcal/100 g. They also contain **potassium**, **iron**, **folic acid** and some **carotene**.

curry A spicy dish of Oriental (particularly Indian) origin, prepared with meat, fish and/or vegetables in a piquant sauce. The nutritional and energy values of curries vary according to the ingredients. The spices, or curry powder, used to give it its characteristic pungent taste are used in such small quantities that they do not affect the nutritional properties of the dish. Very strong (hot) curries may induce sweating.

curry powder A preparation of finely ground pungent spices used to make spicy dishes, especially curry. The spices used vary according to the variety of curry powder, but they usually include **turmeric**, **ginger**, **cumin** and **coriander**. Curry powder is used in such small quantities that it does not affect the nutritional properties of a dish, but strong (hot) curry powder may induce sweating.

custard A hot or cold sweet sauce traditionally made with **eggs**, **milk** and sugar, flavoured with vanilla. Traditional custard provides the nutrients and micronutrients associated with eggs and milk. Custard is now usually made by adding milk (or water and milk) to custard powder, which is predominantly cornflour and sugar; and it may include colouring and flavourings.

cyanocobalamin See **vitamin B₁₂**.

dahl (also called **gram**) A general name for the seeds of certain varieties of leguminous plants (**pulses**) that are mostly cultivated in India, e.g. **mung bean**, **chickpea** and **lentil**. Dahl is also the name given to a spicy dish made from these pulses.

dairy products Any form of **milk** (usually cows' milk), or food derived from milk. There are many different kinds of dairy products and their nutritional and energy values vary. In general they provide **protein**, **sugars** (mostly lactose) and **fat**, with a high proportion of **saturated fatty acids** (if present). Dairy products may be based on full **cream**, semi-skimmed or skimmed milk and will therefore have a variable fat content. With the exception of **butter** they are usually a good source of calcium but other micronutrients will vary according to the product. See also **buttermilk**; **cottage cheese**; **cheese**; **cream cheese**; **crème fraiche**; **curd cheese**; **fromage blanc**; **ghee**; **yoghurt**.

damson The small fruit of a variety of plum tree, with thin, cloudy blue-black skin and crisp, sour yellowish flesh. Damsons are too sour to be eaten fresh and are stewed with sugar or made into jam. They provide **sugars** (as glucose and fructose), **dietary fibre**, very little **protein** and have an energy value of 38 kcal/100 g. They also contain **potassium**, **carotene** and some **vitamin C**. When damsons are stewed with sugar their energy value is increased to 69 kcal/100 g.

dandelion A common Eurasian plant with deeply notched leaves and yellow flowers. Dandelion leaves are added to salads or used to make infusions or wine. The leaves have a high water content and provide some **sugars** and **dietary fibre**. They also contain **potassium**, **iron**, **manganese**, **vitamin C**, **carotene** and **folic acid**, but are eaten in such small amounts that their contribution to the diet is probably negligible. Dandelion infusions may have a mild **laxative** and **diuretic** effect.

date The long, oval fruit of the date palm, with thin, shiny brown skin, crisp, very sweet flesh and a long, woody stone. Dates are eaten fresh or dried, or are used in cakes and desserts. They have a high **sugars** content, provide **dietary fibre**, small amounts of **protein**, and have an energy value of 248 kcal/100 g. They also contain **potassium**, **calcium**, **iron**, **magnesium** and **folic acid**.

decaffeinated A term describing coffee, tea and cola drinks that have had their natural **caffeine** content reduced. Food labelled 'decaffeinated' may still contain small amounts of caffeine (e.g. decaffeinated coffee contains about 4 mg of caffeine per average cup). Only products labelled 'caffeine-free' contain no caffeine.

deep frying A method of cooking where food is wholly immersed in hot fat or oil. Deep frying adds to the energy value of foods because fat is absorbed while the food is cooking. It involves

very high temperatures (180–200°C), and causes
losses of vitamins that are unstable at high temperatures, e.g. **thiamin, pantothenic acid** and **vitamin C**.

dental caries Progressive decay of tooth
enamel that can ultimately lead to the loss of
teeth. Bacteria on the teeth (plaque) metabolize
sugars in food, especially sucrose, and release
lactic acid. The acid gradually breaks down the
enamel and eventually the dentine of the tooth,
causing toothache. Susceptibility to dental caries
can be reduced by good oral hygiene, by reducing
the amount of sugars (especially sucrose) in the
diet and by ensuring an adequate intake of
fluoride.

dextrin A **carbohydrate** produced by the partial
digestion of **starch** before it is broken down to
maltose and ultimately **glucose**; and by the appli-
cation of a dry heat to starch (e.g. toasting bread).
Dextrin forms a sticky gum with water and is used
to thicken foods.

dextrose See **glucose**.

diabetes (diabetes mellitus or **sugar diabetes)**
A disease characterized by an inability to control
blood glucose levels in the body. A lack of the hormone **insulin** or an inability of the body cells to use
insulin properly, causes glucose levels to rise in the
blood (hyperglycaemia) and glucose to spill out in
the urine.

There are two common types of diabetes: insulin-dependent and non-insulin-dependent. In insulin-dependent diabetes, there is insufficient insulin, and regular injections of insulin are necessary to maintain a normal blood glucose level. Non-insulin-dependent diabetes is much more common especially in middle-aged people who are overweight. The condition arises when the body fails to respond to the insulin released by the pancreas. It can usually be controlled by losing weight or by the use of drugs.

Dietary treatment of both types of diabetes is with a diet high in complex **carbohydrates** (starch and dietary fibre) and low in **fat**, **salt** and **sugar**. An overdose of insulin can cause a hypoglycaemic reaction when the blood glucose level falls below normal. Symptoms include hunger, sweating, palpitations, dizziness and mental confusion which are often confused with drunkenness. The blood glucose level should be returned to normal as soon as possible by ingestion of glucose or sucrose. Complications of long-standing diabetes include cataracts, kidney disorders and greater risk of **coronary heart disease**.

diarrhoea A frequent discharge of abnormally liquid faeces, often accompanied by abdominal pain. Diarrhoea may simply be caused by a dietary indiscretion or it can be a symptom of many diseases or disorders including malabsorption diseases, food poisoning, infection, dietary deficiencies or dietary excesses. Fluid intake should be increased to compensate for excessive loss of fluid in the stools. If diarrhoea persists, a doctor should be consulted.

diet The food and drink that a person usually consumes. A balanced diet contains adequate amounts of all nutrients (see the introductory chapter, A BALANCED DIET). A therapeutic diet, devised by a dietitian or doctor, is used to treat many diseases and conditions. Such diets include gluten-free diets for **coeliac disease**, low-protein diets for many kidney diseases and lactose-free diets for **lactose intolerance**. The term is often used to mean a slimming or weight loss diet.

dietary fibre The structural **polysaccharides** of complex **carbohydrates** that are not digested or absorbed in any significant amounts in the body. Dietary fibre is made up of substances that provide the rigid structure to all plants, and it includes **cellulose**, **edible gums** and **pectin**. It does not occur in animals. Some dietary fibre, particularly from **wholegrain** cereals, absorbs water as it passes undigested down the digestive tract and adds bulk and moisture to the stools, encouraging regular and comfortable evacuation of the bowels. Fibre in oats, fruit and vegetables is associated with lowering blood **cholesterol** levels, and preventing a rapid rise in **blood glucose** levels after a meal.

There is no **RDA** for dietary fibre, but a level of 30 g a day is considered desirable. The average UK diet provides only 12 g dietary fibre a day. The best sources of dietary fibre are wholegrain cereals and products made from them including whole-grain breakfast cereals and wholemeal bread, pulses, fruit (particularly dried fruit) and vegetables. Raw bran, particularly wheat bran, is a very rich source of dietary fibre but it is preferable to eat it naturally as part of the wholegrain. Because sudden high intakes of fibre may cause flatulence and distention of the abdomen (this is caused by the fermentation of fibrous matter by intestinal bacteria), dietary fibre should be introduced gradually into the diet. Fluid intake should also be increased because more water is lost in the faeces.

dietary intake The quantity of any **nutrient** or **micronutrient** present in the diet.

dietary requirement The amount of any **nutrient** or **micronutrient** needed in the diet for optimum health. Dietary requirements vary according to age, sex, height, weight and physical activity. Times of physiological stress such as growth in children, pregnancy and lactation increase requirements, as may stress, smoking and alcohol consumption. See also **RDA**.

digestion The bodily process in which foods are broken down into **nutrients**, **protein**, **carbohydrate** and **fat**, and then into their simple component parts for absorption and assimilation. Foods are broken up by chewing and lubricated by saliva in the mouth. In the mouth, stomach and duodenum (the first part of the small intestine), the food is broken down into **amino acids**, **monosaccharides** and **fatty acids** by the actions of the digestive juices. These components as well as vitamins and minerals are absorbed over the huge surface area of the small intestine wall. Undigested and waste matter continues through to the large intestine where some **dietary fibre** may be broken down by intestinal bacteria. Finally the waste matter passes to the rectum and is evacuated through the anus as faeces.

digestive juices The juices secreted in the mouth, stomach and duodenum (the first part of the small intestine) that contain **enzymes** that break down food into its component **amino acids**, **monosaccharides** and **fatty acids**, so that they can be absorbed and assimilated by the body. Enzymes break down specific substances (e.g. amylase breaks starch down to maltose, lactase breaks lactose down to glucose and galactose). Acids and alkalis provide the correct conditions for enyzmes to function. **Bile**, formed in the liver and stored in the gall bladder, emulsifies the fat so that it can be digested. In some conditions the synthesis or function of certain digestive juices may be impaired, such as **lactose intolerance** or **coeliac disease**.

dill The leaves and seed-like fruits of a Eurasian shrub that are used fresh or dried to give flavour to foods, especially pickles. Dill is used in such small quantities that its nutritional properties are negligible.

disaccharide Simple **carbohydrates** or **sugars** consisting of two monosaccharides joined together. Disaccharides include **sucrose**, **maltose** and **lactose**. They are broken down by enzymes in the digestive tract to their constituent monosaccharides, which are then absorbed and carried in the blood to the liver for energy supply.

diuretic A substance that increases the flow of urine. Diuretics are used to control **oedema**, which can be caused by certain heart, liver and kidney complaints. Overuse of diuretics can cause dehydration and may leach the body of certain micronutrients, especially **potassium**. **Caffeine** is a naturally occurring diuretic.

dried fruit Any kind of fruit (e.g. apricots, figs, grapes and plums) allowed to mature and dry on the tree, but is now usually artificially dried. Because they have a low water content, dried fruits are – weight for weight – a richer source of the nutrients and minerals than fresh fruit. They are usually high in **dietary fibre** (especially dried figs and prunes) and have high **sugars** contents, and correspondingly high energy values. Most vitamins are also concentrated in dried fruit, but **vitamin C** and **biotin** are lost altogether. See **prunes**; **raisins**; **sultanas**.

drinking chocolate A powder of cocoa and sugar to which hot or cold milk (or water and milk) is added to make a drink. It is also used to flavour biscuits, cakes and desserts. Chocolate powder contains neither of the stimulants, **caffeine** and theobromine, found in cocoa. It has a high **sugars** content, contains some **fat** with a high proportion of **saturated fatty acids**, some **protein** and has an energy value of 366 kcal/100 g. It contains small amounts of **potassium**, **sodium**, **magnesium**, **iron**, **copper**, **zinc**, **chloride** and **folic acid**.

dripping The fat that seeps from meat when it is roasting and is often gathered and used for cooking. Dripping is 99% fat with a high proportion of **saturated fatty acids**, a correspondingly high energy value of 891 kcal/100 g and negligible amounts of any micronutrients.

duck The rich, fatty meat of an aquatic bird that may be domesticated (poultry) or shot as **game**. Duck provides **protein** and **fat**, much of which is in the skin. Removing the skin before or after cooking reduces the fat content considerably, and reduces the energy value from 339 kcal/100 g (roasted) to 189 kcal/100 g (roasted). Duck contains **potassium**, **phosphorus**, **iron**, **zinc**, **sulphur**, **niacin**, **vitamin B$_{12}$**, **folic acid**, **pantothenic acid** and **biotin**.

dyspepsia Indigestion, including **heartburn**. It can also refer to the general discomfort and dis-

tension sometimes felt after a meal. Dyspepsia can
be a symptom of a digestive disorder such as
peptic **ulcer** or **hiatus hernia**.

eczema A non-contagious but possibly hereditary inflammation of the skin. It is characterized
by dry, scaly, itching patches, especially in the
elbows and behind the knees. If the lesions are
scratched, they form painful, weeping scabs.
Eczema can be brought on or aggravated by emotional stress or by food allergies. Dietary treatment involves removal of the food or foods
causing a reaction, usually cows' milk, eggs, beef
and chicken, but many other foods have been
implicated. Eczema is a common condition in
infancy and it is important that the diet remains
balanced and supports optimum growth while
eliminating the reactive foods.

edible gum A complex **carbohydrate** that has a
gum-like structure. It is extracted from tree sap
(e.g. gum arabic) and from seeds (e.g. guar and
carob gums). Edible gums are not digested but
add to the **dietary fibre** intake. They lower blood
cholesterol levels and prevent a rapid rise in **blood
glucose** levels after a meal. Edible gums are used as
food additives, as emulsifiers, stabilizers and
thickeners.

egg The mature ovum of a hen (or other poultry), protected by a calcified shell. Eggs are eaten
boiled, fried, baked, or scrambled with milk and

are used extensively in cooking. Eggs provide **protein** and are a rich source of **cholesterol**. All the **fat** is concentrated in the yolk and it contains a high proportion of **saturated fatty acids**. Eggs contain **sodium**, **potassium**, **phosphorus**, poorly-absorbed **iron**, **zinc**, **sulphur**, **retinol**, **vitamin D**, **niacin**, **vitamin E**, **pantothenic acid**, **biotin**, **folic acid** and **vitamin B$_{12}$**. Free-range eggs contain slightly more **vitamin B$_{12}$** than battery eggs. Most of the nutritional value of eggs is in the yolk. A substance in egg-white inhibits the absorption of biotin, unless it is properly cooked. None of the **micronutrients** are seriously depleted when eggs are cooked.

eggplant See **aubergine**.

endive The loosely packed, leafy bud of a European plant, eaten in salads. Endives have a high water content, provide small amounts of **dietary fibre**, **protein** and **sugars**, and have an energy value of 11 kcal/100 g. They are a good source of **carotene**, **folic acid** and **iron**.

energy The capacity of a body to do work. A constant energy supply is essential for all bodily processes, e.g. digestion, physical activity, growth and repairing tissues. It is supplied from food and released by breaking down the major food components, **fat**, **sugars**, **carbohydrate** and **protein** (as well as **alcohol**). See also **energy requirement**; **energy value of food**.

energy requirement The amount of energy needed by the body for maintenance and activity

91

while keeping a constant body weight. The energy requirement of an individual varies according to their age, sex, height, weight and physical activity. Energy requirements are usually expressed in terms of heat and measured in **joules** or **calories**. If the energy requirement is greater than the energy provided by the diet, the body's energy stores of **glycogen** and then **fat** are used to make up the difference. If the energy requirement is less than the energy provided by the diet, the excess energy in the form of **carbohydrate**, fat and **protein** is converted to body fat and stored.

energy value of food   The amount of energy provided by **protein**, **fat** and **carbohydrate** in food. Energy values are usually expressed in terms of heat and are measured in kilojoules or kilocalories (kcal) per 100 g of the food or drink. One gram of dietary carbohydrate provides 4 kcal, one gram of fat provides 9 kcal, and one gram of protein provides 4 kcal.

E number   A classification of a food **additive**. It was adopted by the European Communities to provide a simple and concise way of referring to those additives that are on the permitted lists of every EC country. Those additives with only a number and no E are on the permitted lists of some but not all EC countries.

enzyme   A **protein** made in the body to catalyse the body's chemical reactions, such as digestion and metabolism. Each enzyme performs a specific function, e.g. lipase breaks down **fat** into **fatty acids**, sucrase breaks down **sucrose** into **glucose** and **fructose**, and trypsin breaks down **protein** into **peptides** and **amino acids**.

essential oil   One of a number of volatile, usually highly perfumed substances (not in fact a **lipid**) that are extracted from parts of plants (usually nuts and kernels) and used as flavouring or for their medicinal properties, e.g. almond oil is used to give flavour to biscuits, cakes and pastries, and oil of cloves is traditionally used to alleviate toothache.

eucalyptus oil   A fragrant **essential oil** extracted from the leaves of the eucalyptus tree and valued for its disinfectant properties. Eucalyptus oil is one of the principal ingredients in some kinds of mouthwash and toothpaste.

evening primrose oil   The oil extracted from the seeds of the evening primrose. It is rich in **polyunsaturated fatty acids**, with a high proportion of **linoleic acid** and **gamma-linolenic acid**. Evening primrose oil as a supplement may be beneficial in soothing **eczema**, or other skin conditions, when applied locally or taken in capsules. It is reported by some women to alleviate the uncomfortable abdominal pains associated with premenstrual syndrome.

ewes' milk   The milk of the female sheep. It has a similar nutritional value to cows' milk but with a higher **fat**, **protein** and energy value. Ewes' milk is sometimes tolerated by those allergic to the protein in cows' milk. Ewes' milk is used to make a strong, fatty French cheese called Roquefort.

extrusion cooking   A method of cooking a food as it is extruded. The food in the form of a paste is forced through holes in a plate and then cooked immediately. Extrusion cooking is used in making pasta, snack foods, many breakfast cereals and **textured vegetable protein**.

factory farming (or **intensive farming**)   A method of farming in which animals are intensively reared using modern industrial methods. Factory farming produces food efficiently and inexpensively, particularly meat, eggs and milk. It has little effect on the nutritient content of the food. However, it is increasingly considered that factory farming methods of feeding and raising animals promote the spread of disease, such as salmonella in chickens and BSE in cattle. Many conscientious shoppers avoid factory-farmed products for ethical reasons, preferring to buy food that has been farmed in a more traditional way.

fast food   Any kind of food that has been pre-prepared and can be quickly cooked and eaten with a minimum of effort. The nutritional and energy values of fast foods vary considerably, but in general they have a high **fat** and **sugars** content, and a correspondingly high energy value. Savouries tend to be highly salted, and have a high **sodium** content. Many forms of fast food are prepared using food **additives**.

fats Large organic compounds that are insoluble in water and are found in the body as body fat, and as a nutrient in food with a very high energy value. Fats are made up of **triglycerides**, compounds of **glycerol** and **fatty acids**. The body can make fat from **carbohydrate** and **protein**, only requiring essential fatty acids to be supplied in the diet. Fat-free diets, in which most of the energy is supplied by carbohydrate, tend to be bulky because fat is such a concentrated source of energy in the diet. Foods with very high fat contents are vegetable oils, dripping, lard, butter, margarine, cream, nuts and some meats. Bacon and lamb have a high fat content, but it can be reduced by trimming the visible fat before or after cooking. As fat is a concentrated source of energy, a high fat intake can lead to excessive levels of energy and an increase in body weight, leading to **overweight** and **obesity**. High intakes of fat, particularly fats with a high proportion of **saturated fatty acids**, are associateard with increased risk of **coronary heart disease** and cancer (particularly of the breast). See also the introductory chapter, A BALANCED DIET.

fatty acids Organic compounds that contain a chemical group known as an acid group, and which are usually joined with **glycerol** to form **triglycerides**. There are three kinds of fatty acids: **saturated**, unsaturated and **polyunsaturated**. These classifications are determined by the number of hydrogen units that are missing. Saturated fatty acids have none missing, polyunsaturated fatty acids have four or more missing. Two families of polyunsaturated fatty acids, the **linoleic acid** and alpha-linolenic acid families, are essential as they cannot be made in the body and must be obtained from the diet. Essential fatty acids (EFA) are important components of cell membranes, the sheath that protects nerves and some hormones. The diet should contain sufficient fat in order to ensure the intake of EFAs. The best sources of EFAs are safflower-seed oil, evening primrose oil, sunflower oil, soya bean oil and corn oil.

EFA deficiency is first indicated by dry, scaly skin and poor hair condition. Polyunsaturated fatty acids are important in maintaining correct blood **cholesterol** levels. They actively lower the level and reduce susceptibility to **atherosclerosis** and **coronary heart disease**, but their effect is not as great as that of saturated fatty acids in raising blood cholesterol levels. To reduce the risk of heart disease, the total fat intake should be reduced, particularly the saturated fatty acid intake, and a greater proportion of the reduced fat intake should be fat with a high proportion of polyunsaturated fatty acids.

fennel The crisp, fibrous, strong-smelling stem

of a shrub that is eaten raw in salads or boiled and eaten as a vegetable. Fennel has a high water content, provides some **dietary fibre**, small amounts of **sugars** and **protein**, and has an energy value of 28 kcal/100 g. It also contains **potassium**, some **folic acid** and **vitamin C**. Much of the folic acid and vitamin C are lost when it is boiled.

fennel seed The dried seed of fennel, used to add flavour to food, especially fish. Fennel seeds are used in such small quantities that their nutritional properties are negligible.

fenugreek The dried seeds of a heavily scented, Mediterranean leguminous plant that are dried and used to flavour food. Fenugreek is used in such small quantities that its nutritional properties are negligible.

fermentation A chemical reaction in which a substance (e.g. yeast, mould, bacteria or enzymes) breaks down an organic molecule into simpler components. For example, in the making of alcoholic drinks, **yeast** ferments **sugars** to give alcohol; in digestion intestinal bacteria ferment some types of **dietary fibre**, releasing gas, which causes flatulence.

fertilizer Any substance added to soil to increase its crop yield. Fertilizers include natural substances, e.g. manure and compost, and artificial substances such as nitrates (see **nitrate** and nitrite). Fertilizers may still be present in foods, principally plants but also animals fed with fertilized fodder. Some of the chemicals used in fertilizers could be harmful if they were consumed in large quantities. Foods that have not been treated with fertilizers, or **insecticides**, are called **organic foods**.

fibre See **dietary fibre**.

fig The pear-shaped fruit-pod of a tropical and sub-tropical tree. It has smooth, fleshy, green or purple skin with sweet, pinkish flesh and many tiny seed-like fruits. Figs provide **sugars**, **dietary fibre**, some **protein** and have an energy value of 41 kcal/100 g. They also contain **potassium**, **carotene** and some **vitamin C**. Dried figs are a good source of dietary fibre, provide **potassium**, some **calcium** and **iron**, but only a little **carotene** and no vitamin C. They have an energy value of 213 kcal/100 g. If figs are stewed or preserved in syrup, most of the carotene and all of the vitamin C are lost.

fish Any species of edible marine or fresh-water aquatic vertebra. Edible fish fall into two categories: white fish, which contain very little fat (less than 3%), and fatty fish, which have moderate to high fat contents (with a high proportion of essential **polyunsaturated fatty acids**). The nutritional properties and energy values of fish vary, but in general they provide **protein**, many minerals and **B complex vitamins**. Fatty fish contain **vitamin A** and

vitamin D. Some fish are eaten whole, including
the bones, and are therefore a good source of **calcium**. When fish is fried, the fat content and energy
value are increased considerably. See **anchovy**;
cod; **haddock**, **halibut**; **herring**; **kipper**; **mackerel**;
mullet; **pilchard**; **plaice**; **rollmop**; **saithe**; **salmon**;
sardine; **skate**; **sole**; **sprat**; **trout**; **tuna**; **whitebait**;
whiting. See also **shellfish**; **roe**; **caviar**.

flatulence An excessive amount of gas in the
digestive tract, that may cause uncomfortable distension of the abdomen and may be expelled
through the mouth or anus. Flatulence in the
stomach is usually caused by swallowing air
(caused by eating too quickly or talking while
eating) and in the intestine by gas released during
the fermentation of some types of **dietary fibre** by
intestinal bacteria.

flour Finely ground cereals, especially wheat,
used in making bread, biscuits, pasta, cakes,
pastry and many other foods. Flour is an important basic ingredient and a major source of **carbohydrate** and energy in the diet. Wholegrain or
wholemeal wheat flour provides **starch**, **dietary
fibre**, **protein**, small amounts of **sugars** and **fat**, and
has an energy value of 318 kcal/100 g. It also contains **potassium**, **magnesium**, **phosphorus**, **iron**,
zinc, some **vitamin E** and most of the **B complex
vitamins**, (particularly niacin, folic acid and
biotin). Brown flour has had some of the bran
removed and provides more starch and less diet-

ary fibre and micronutrients. White flour is highly refined and contains no bran. It has a much higher starch content and provides little dietary fibre and contains only very small amounts of the above micronutrients. Brown and white flour are legally fortified with thiamin, niacin, iron and calcium to a minimum level that matches the amounts found in wholegrain flour. Flour may be made from other cereals, and its nutritional value varies according to the cereal used.

fluoride A non-metallic essential **trace element**, found mostly in the teeth and bones. Fluoride helps children to develop strong bones and teeth, and protects teeth from **dental caries**. There is no **RDA** for fluoride, but it is generally accepted that the average daily intake of 1–3 mg is adequate for adults. The best sources of fluoride are tea and seaweeds. It is also naturally present in drinking water, and added during water treament. Fluoride deficiency increases susceptibility to dental caries and causes weak teeth and bones in children. Fluoride is toxic in excess and causes degeneration of tooth enamel (indicated by discolouring and pitting of the teeth) and, ultimately, the bones.

folic acid One of the **B complex vitamins**. It is supplied in the diet but is also made in the body by intestinal bacteria. Folic acid is involved in the synthesis of **amino acids** and of the chemical groups in genes that pass on genetic information, and in the production of blood. There is no UK

RDA for folic acid, but the US RDA is 400 µg. Requirements are increased during pregnancy and lactation (see APPENDIX II, SPECIAL NEEDS). The best sources are leafy green vegetables, liver, pulses, eggs, wholemeal cereal products, brewer's yeast, wheatgerm and wheat bran. Much of the folic acid content of foods can be lost in cooking and processing because it is unstable at high temperatures and is easily **leached** into cooking water. In the body it is depleted by some drugs, including the contraceptive pill. A deficiency of folic acid causes a form of **anaemia**.

food additives   See **additives**.

food allergy   See **allergy (food)**.

food fortification (also called **food enrichment**) The addition of nutrients, particularly vitamins, minerals and sometimes amino acids to foods in order to improve their nutritional value. Manufacturers are bound by law to enrich some products, e.g. margarine is fortified with vitamin A and vitamin D (in order to match the quantities of these vitamins in butter), and white and brown flour are enriched with niacin, thiamin, iron and calcium (in order to compensate for the losses of these micronutrients when flour is refined).

food labelling   The system of clearly identifying foods and their ingredients on labels. Manufacturers are bound by law to name all the ingredients in their products, and this includes any additives that may have been used. These must be listed strictly in order by weight, i.e. those that are present in most significant amounts appear first. The label should also state a date before which the food must be eaten. If a 'sell-by' date is shown, it should also give some indication of how soon the product should be eaten after purchase or after opening.

food poisoning Acute illness caused by foods or substances in them, and characterized by pains in the stomach and abdomen, vomiting and diarrhoea. There are many different causes of food poisoning: bacteria (e.g. **salmonella**), moulds (e.g. **aflatoxins**), chemicals (e.g. **mercury**) and toxic substances that occur naturally in foods (e.g. **lectins**). Food poisoning can be fatal, particularly in susceptible groups such as babies, young children and the elderly. A doctor should always be consulted if food poisoning is suspected.

food preservation Any method of treating food in order to arrest decomposition, prolong its shelf-life and minimize the risk of food poisoning. Food may be preserved by the addition of salt (e.g. in cured meats), sugar (e.g. in jam or crystallized fruit), vinegar (e.g. in pickles) or other, often chemical, preservatives. It may also be treated in a number of ways to destroy bacteria or arrest their activities, e.g. freezing, canning, cooking, smoking, vacuum-packing, irradiating or refrigeration.

Many methods of preservation cause losses of vitamins and minerals, especially vitamin C and folic acid, and further losses occur (especially of carotene and vitamin C) if preserved foods are stored for a long time.

food processing Any treatment given to food to prepare it for eating and in some cases for packaging and storage, including peeling, chopping, refining, cooking and preserving. Most forms of food processing cause some losses of micronutrients, and many forms, e.g. refining cereals and peeling fruits and vegetables, reduce the dietary fibre content of foods.

food spoilage The decomposition of food either by bacteria or by enzymes that are present in the food itself. Food spoilage is reduced by **food preservation** and can be further arrested if foods are kept dry and/or refrigerated or are stored according to manufacturers' instructions. Shoppers should check the labels on food to see when the product should be consumed. If food is eaten when it has started to decompose, it can cause food poisoning.

food supplement See **supplement**.

French bean The slender, green seed pods of a small, twining leguminous plant, an immature **pulse**. French beans are usually boiled and eaten as vegetables, or they may be **parboiled** and used cold in salads. They have a high water content, provide small amounts of **dietary fibre**, **sugars**, **protein** and **starch**, and have an energy value of 35 kcal/100 g. They also contain **carotene** and **folic acid**, and small amounts of **iron** and **vitamin C**. The folic acid and vitamin C contents are reduced when they are cooked. Even though the seeds are immature, like all pulses, they may contain **phytic acid** and **lectins**, and they should be cooked in order to destroy these substances.

fromage blanc (also called **fromage frais**) A smooth, fluid, white cheese made by fermenting skimmed milk, and often used as a low-fat substitute for cream in cooking and on fruit. Fromage blanc provides high-quality **protein** and small amounts of **sugars**. It is valued for its low **fat** content (shoppers should check labels, which indicate what percentage of fromage blanc is fat, usually 0%, 20% or 40%, and the corresponding energy value). It also contains **phosphorus**, **retinol**, **carotene**, **niacin** and **folic acid**. Unlike other cheeses, fromage blanc is not made with salt, and it has a low **sodium** content.

fromage frais See **fromage blanc**.

frozen food Foods that have been **blanched** to destroy active **enzymes**, and then kept at a steady sub-zero temperature (usually –18°C) to preserve them. Freezing is a good method of food preservation because it does not entail great losses of vitamins. Some vitamins that are unstable at high temperatures (e.g. **vitamin C** and **pantothenic acid**) may be lost during **blanching**, and there may be further losses of these two vitamins and of vitamin E when frozen foods are stored. When frozen foods are thawed small amounts of the water-soluble vitamins (the **B complex vitamins** and **vitamin C**) may be **leached** into the water, and this water should be used with the food to minimize these losses.

fructose A **monosaccharide** or simple sugar found in honey and in most fruit, and with another monosaccharide, **glucose**, forms the disaccharide **sucrose**. Fructose is absorbed more slowly than glucose and does not cause a rapid rise in **blood glucose** levels. It is sometimes used in the dietary treatment of **diabetics**.

fruit The fleshy, ripened ovary of a plant, containing one or more seeds. Some fruits are eaten as vegetables, e.g. tomatoes and marrows, but most are eaten as fruit, i.e. by themselves or in desserts. The nutritional and energy values of fruits vary enormously, but in general they have a high water content and provide **sugars** (mostly fructose and glucose), **dietary fibre**, some **starch**, small amounts of **protein** and no **fat**. Most fruits provide **vitamin C** and **carotene**. Many fruits are available canned, containing less vitamin C and carotene than fresh fruits, and if they are canned in syrup they have higher energy values. See **apple**; **apricot**; **banana**;

blackberry; blackcurrant; cherry; citrus fruit; damson; date; fig; greengage; grape; guava; kiwi fruit; loganberry; lychee; mango; nectarine; papaya; peach; pineapple; raspberry; strawberry. See also **dried fruit**; **fruit juice**.

fruit juice The juice extracted from fruit. The nutritional and energy values of fruit juices vary according to the fruit from which they are extracted. In general they provide **sugars** and some of the micronutrients associated with fruit, e.g. vitamin C and vitamin A. Some fruit juices may contain added sugar, and some may contain additives such as artificial colourings.

fruitarian A person who eats only fruit, nuts and seeds. Such diets can result in **anaemia**, weight loss through inadequate energy intake and vitamin deficiencies.

frying A method of cooking in a small amount of very hot oil or fat (compare to **deep frying**). Frying adds to the energy value of foods because some of the fat is absorbed, it also causes heavy losses of vitamins that are unstable at high temperatures, e.g. vitamin C and pantothenic acid.

fungi A group of simple plants that do not synthesize food using sunlight, including mushrooms, toadstools, moulds and yeast. Many species are edible but few are eaten in the UK.

fungicide See **pesticide**.

galactose A **monosaccharide** chiefly found combined with **glucose** to form **lactose**. Galactose is absorbed into the bloodstream following lactose digestion and is then normally converted into glucose in the liver.

game Any animal, or bird, that is shot for sport and eaten. All game, with the exception of **pigeon** and **rabbit**, is protected by law and has a closed season when it may not be shot or sold. Game may be bred specially for shooting or it may even be reared and slaughtered like other livestock. The nutritional properties and energy values of game vary enormously because it includes birds, small mammals and larger animals, such as deer. See **duck**; **grouse**; **hare**; **partridge**; **pheasant**; **quail**; **venison**.

gamma-linolenic acid A **polyunsaturated fatty acid**, a longer chain derivative of the essential fatty acid **linoleic acid**, that is produced in the body. Individual differences in the ability to form gamma-linolenic acid may have important implications for a variety of disorders. Very few foods contain gamma-linolenic acid, although **evening primrose oil** contains large amounts and may be taken as a supplement.

gammon The cured leg of a pig, usually the fore-leg (the hind-leg is used for **hams**). Gammon may be smoked or unsmoked (green) and is usually roasted or boiled. It provides **protein** and has a fairly high **fat** content, and a correspondingly high energy value of 239 kcal/100 g. The fat content can be reduced by trimming away visible fat before or after cooking. Gammon also contains **potassium**, **phosphorus**, **zinc** and **niacin** as well as some **iron**, **thiamin** and **biotin**. Some of the potassium and thiamin are lost if it is boiled. It is heavily salted and has a very high **sodium** content.

garden pea See **pea**.

garlic The pungent bulb of a small Asian plant, divided into many separate 'cloves', used fresh or dried and powdered to give flavour to food. Garlic is used more for its flavour properties than for its nutritional value. It has also been used and valued since ancient times to aid digestion and as a mild disinfectant for the digestive system. Garlic in large daily doses (30 g) has been shown to reduce the level of blood **cholesterol**, but the mechanism is not yet understood.

gelatin A **protein** formed from collagen (a cementing substance that binds cells together). It is manufactured commercially from hide, skin and bones. Alhough soluble in water, in sufficient concentrations it forms a solid jelly when it cools and is used as the basis of sweet jellies and aspic. Gelatin is a poor-quality protein because it contains none of the essential **amino acid** tryptophan and little phenylalanine.

ghee Clarified butter, a clear, yellow liquid obtained by heating butter so that the fat melts, the water is evaporated and the milk solids can be skimmed off. Ghee is traditionally used in Indian cooking. It has an exceptionally high energy value of 910 kcal/100 g, a high saturated **fatty acid** content and provides small amounts of **vitamin A** and **vitamin D**. If it is made with salted butter it has a high **sodium** content.

gherkin A very small cucumber grown for pickling and preserved in vinegar. Used mostly for garnishes and savoury snacks, it does not provide significant amounts of any **nutrients** or **micronutrients**.

gin An alcoholic drink obtained from distilling barley grains and flavoured with juniper berries. Gin usually contains approximately 40% alcohol by volume. It has a high energy value of 222 kcal/100 g (three measures), but it is deficient in all other nutrients.

ginger The spicy, pungent underground stem of an Indian plant that is used fresh or dried and powdered to give flavour to foods, especially curries, biscuits and cakes. Ginger may also be crystallized in sugar or preserved in syrup and eaten as a delicacy or added to foods. As a spice, it is used in such small quantities that its nutritional properties are negligible. The crystallized stems or stems in syrup contain large amounts of **sugars** and have correspondingly high energy values of 214 kcal/100 g (drained). They also provide small amounts of **starch** and **dietary fibre**, **magnesium**, **iron**, **manganese** and **zinc**.

ginger ale   A sweet, carbonated drink, flavoured with **ginger** and used as a mixer with spirits. Ginger ale provides **sugars** and has an energy value of approximately 25 kcal/100 ml (reduced-calorie ginger ale is also available). It does not provide significant amounts of any other nutrients and it may contain colouring and flavouring.

ginger beer   A mild, spicy and slightly effervescent alcoholic drink obtained by distilling sugars and stem **ginger**. Ginger beer contains 5% **alcohol** by volume, some **sugars** (reduced-calorie ginger beer is also available) and has an energy value of 35 kcal/100 g. It does not provide significant amounts of any other nutrients and it may contain colouring and flavouring.

ginseng   The forked aromatic root of several varieties of Asian plant (usually from China or Korea). The Chinese traditionally use it fresh or dried and powdered for medicinal purposes. Ginseng is available in infusions, capsules or as a powder. Although the Chinese have used it for centuries as a cure and a restorative for a number of complaints its effectiveness has not been proven or explained, but it remains a popular dietary supplement.

globe artichoke   The large thistle-like flower head of a tall Asian plant. It has large, tough

petals that have a pleasant tasting fleshy base, and
a smooth, fleshy edible 'heart'. Immature artichokes may be eaten raw or the mature flower
head may be boiled and the fleshy part at its base
eaten. They have a high water content, provide
only very small amounts of **protein** and have an
energy value of 15 kcal/100 g. Globe artichokes
contain good amounts of **potassium** and **calcium**
but few other micronutrients. Globe artichokes
are usually served with butter or oily dressings
which will increase the fat content and energy
value.

glucose (also called **dextrose**, **grape sugar** and
blood sugar) A **monosaccharide** or simple
sugar. Glucose occurs naturally in honey and
grapes and as part of the disaccharide **sucrose** and
polysaccharide **starch**. It can be made in the body
from **protein** and **fat**, and is manufactured commercially from starch by the action of acid or
enzymes. During digestion **carbohydrate** is broken
down into glucose, which is absorbed into the
blood and carried to the liver. It is either used
immediately for energy or converted into **glycogen**
or **fat** and stored. Glucose has the same energy
value as other sugars and starch, although it is half
as sweet as sucrose. See **blood glucose**.

glucose syrup A sugary liquid, resulting from
the partial breakdown of **starch**, usually maize or
corn. It is a mixture of **glucose**, **maltose** and several
complex sugars, but glucose is the sugar present in

111

the highest concentrations. Glucose syrup is less sweet than glucose and it is used particularly in confectionery and soft drinks. It has a similar energy value to other sugars and starch.

gluten A **protein** found predominantly in wheat and rye. It is the presence of gluten in wheat and rye that makes these cereals suitable for making leavened **bread**. When the dough is kneaded the gluten becomes elastic and expands, it traps the carbon dioxide given off by yeast fermentation. Other cereals, such as barley, maize, millet, oats and rice, either contain none or insufficient to make bread. A gluten-free diet is used as part of the treatment of **coeliac disease**.

glycogen A **polysaccharide** of **glucose** units, synthesized and stored in the liver and muscles for energy supply. The store is small and in starvation is used up in about 24 hours. Liver glycogen is broken down into glucose, which is used to keep a constant **blood glucose** concentration. Muscle glycogen is also broken down into glucose, which can then be used to supply muscles with energy for movement. The muscle glycogen levels can be increased by eating a diet high in **carbohydrate**, and this can be particularly beneficial for endurance athletes (see APPENDIX II, SPECIAL NEEDS).

goats' cheese The tangy, pungent cheese made from goats' milk. The nutritional properties of goats' cheese are similar to cheese made from cows' milk. Goat cheeses provide **protein**, variable amounts of **fat** and **saturated fatty acids**, and have correspondingly variable energy values. They are rich in **calcium**, **vitamin A** and **riboflavin** and may contain added salt and have a high **sodium** content. Goats' cheese is sometimes tolerated by those allergic to the protein in cows' milk.

goats' milk The milk of the goat. It has a similar nutritional content to cows' milk except it has a higher **fat** and lower **folic acid** content. Goats' milk is sometimes tolerated by those allergic to the protein in cows' milk. Unlike cows' milk, the production and handling of goats' milk is not covered by regulations and because of the risk of infection, goats' milk should be boiled before use.

goose The rich, fatty flesh of the goose, a domestic poultry bird. Goose provides **protein**, **fat** and has an energy value of 319 kcal/100 g (roast). Much of the fat is in the skin and the fat content and energy value can be reduced if the skin is removed before or after cooking. Goose is a good source of **iron** and it contains small amounts of **calcium** and **magnesium**.

gooseberry The pale green or deep red, many-seeded fruit of a small, spiny Eurasian shrub. Large, sweet dessert gooseberries contain more **sugars** than the cooking varieties, although sugar may be added in cooking. Gooseberries have a high water content and provide only very small amounts of **dietary fibre** and **protein**. They also contain **potassium** and **carotene** (more in red varieties). Gooseberries are a good source of **vitamin C**, which is not lost on cooking and canning due to the high acidity of gooseberries. Dessert varieties have an energy value of 37 kcal/100 g and cooking varieties stewed with sugar of 50 kcal/100 g.

gout A localized and recurrent form of **arthritis**, causing painful inflammation usually of the big toe and finger joints. Gout results from the accumulation of uric acid crystals in the joints. Uric acid is a waste product of purines, substances found in offal, yeast and yeast extracts, roes and some fish and meat. Gout is treated with drugs, but diet is helpful in reducing the number of attacks. Excessive fat and foods that are rich in purines should be avoided and an acceptable body weight maintained. See also APPENDIX I, LOSING AND GAINING WEIGHT.

gram See **dahl**.

grape The pale green ('white') or deep red ('black') fruits of the vine, which grow in clusters and have thin skins, smooth juicy flesh and small, bitter, woody seeds. Dessert grapes are usually eaten fresh, and many varieties are used to make wine. They contain **sugars** and very small amounts of **dietary fibre** and **protein**. White grapes have an energy value of 63 kcal/100 g and black grapes a value of 61 kcal/100 g. Grapes also contain **potas-**

sium, manganese (more in black varieties than in white), **folic acid** (more in white varieties than in black) and some **vitamin C**. See also **raisins; sultanas**.

grapefruit A large citrus fruit with shiny, waxy yellow skin, juicy flesh in crescent-shaped segments and small woody pips. Grapefruits provide **sugars** and only very small amounts of **dietary fibre** and **protein**. They are reliable sources of **vitamin C** and also contain **potassium**, **folic acid** and small amounts of **biotin**. Some of the potassium, vitamin C and folic acid are lost if they are cooked or canned. Grapefruits have low energy values of 22 kcal/100 g, but their energy value is raised if they are canned in syrup or served with sugar.

gravy The juices from roasting meat, which form a sediment and once the fat is poured off are diluted with stock or vegetable cooking water. Gravy may also be thickened with flour and coloured with caramel (gravy browning). Some of the minerals and vitamins **leached** out during cooking are recovered in the gravy. The nutritional and energy values depend very much on the ingredients used. Commercially produced gravy granules have a high **sodium** content, and they may contain **monosodium glutamate** and flavouring and colouring.

greengage A small fruit of a variety of plum, with thin green skin, sweet juicy yellowish flesh and a hard stone. Greengages provide **sugars**, small amounts of **dietary fibre** and **protein**, and have an energy value of 47 kcal/100 g and 75 kcal/ 100 g when stewed with sugar. They contain **potassium** but very little **vitamin C**.

grilling A method of cooking by radiant heat, using electricity, gas or charcoal. Grilling causes the outside of the food to reach high temperatures (above 100°C) and may cause some losses of vitamins that are unstable at high temperatures, e.g. **thiamin** and **pantothenic acid**. Minerals and vitamins may be **leached** into the juices that escape from food during cooking, but grilling lowers the fat content and energy value as fat drips out under the intense heat. Grilling preserves the natural flavour of food better than any other methods but it is not suitable for tough cuts of meat because it further toughens the meat fibres.

groundnuts See **peanuts**.

groundnut oil The vegetable oil extracted from groundnuts (peanuts), which is used for cooking and dressings. Groundnut oil contains a high proportion of monounsaturated **fatty acids**, has an energy value of 899 kcal/100 g and is rich in **vitamin E**.

grouse A game bird. Grouse provides **protein**, is low in **fat** and has an energy value of 173 kcal/100 g. It is rich in well-absorbed **iron** and also contains **potassium**, **calcium** and **magnesium**.

guar gum An **edible gum** extracted from the seeds of an Asian plant. As a food additive it is used as a thickening agent and stabilizer, particularly in sauces and ice cream. Like other edible gums, it is not digested but contributes to **dietary fibre** intake. It has been shown to lower blood **cholesterol** and **blood glucose** levels, and is sometimes used in the treatment of **diabetes**.

guava The small fruit of a tropical American tree, with yellow skin and pulpy, sweet pink flesh. Guavas may be eaten fresh or canned or they may be used to make jam. They provide **sugars**, small amounts of **dietary fibre** and **protein**, and have an energy value of 57 kcal/100 g. They are a particularly good source of **vitamin C** and only small amounts are lost in canning.

haggis A traditional Scottish dish made with offal (usually sheep or calf), oats and suet tightly packed into a skin made from the animal's stomach, and boiled. The nutritional properties and energy values of haggis depend on the exact ingredients, but in general it provides some **protein**, **starch** and **fat** with a high proportion of **saturated fatty acids**, and an energy value of 310 kcal/100 g. It is rich in **retinol** and **biotin**, and also contains **potassium**, **phosphorus**, **iron**, **zinc**, **niacin**, **vitamin B$_{12}$** and **folic acid**. It is usually salted and therefore has a high **sodium** content.

haddock An Atlantic white fish, similar to **cod**, but smaller and with a stronger flavour. Haddock

117

may be eaten poached, steamed, baked, fried,
deep fried or cooked in the microwave; it is also
available smoked. It provides **protein**, very little
fat and has an energy value of 98 kcal/100 g
(fresh). The fat content and energy value are
increased when haddock is fried. It also contains
**potassium, phosphorus, sulphur, niacin, vitamin
B₁₂, folic acid, biotin** and some **iron**. Frying and
smoking destroy some of the niacin and all of the
vitamin B₁₂, folic acid and biotin. Smoked haddock has a very high **sodium** content.

hair Threads of toughened dead cells that grow
from tiny glands under the skin. Hair condition
can be an indicator of general health, and some
dietary deficiencies may be indicated by loss of
condition in the hair, especially **trace elements**
such as **zinc** and **B complex vitamin** deficiencies.
Hair loss can also be due to excess **vitamin A** and
niacin.

halibut An Atlantic white fish with dense meaty
flesh. Halibut is the largest flat fish eaten, and is
usually served poached, steamed or baked. It provides **protein** and very little **fat**. It also contains
potassium, phosphorus, sulphur, niacin, folic acid
and **biotin**, and some **vitamin E** and **vitamin B₁₂**.
None of these micronutrients is seriously depleted
when it is cooked.

ham The hind-leg of a pig specially cured and
usually smoked. However, the word ham is used

to mean a variety of different cuts of cured pig meat, and it is available fresh, tinned or sliced and vacuum-packed, and is usually eaten cold. The nutritional properties and energy values of ham vary according to the cut; in general it provides **protein** and some saturated **fat** (the fat content can be reduced by trimming the visible fat); it also contains **potassium, phosphorus, niacin, iron, thiamin** and **biotin** (much of the thiamin is lost in canned ham). All ham is highly salted and has a high **sodium** content. To reduce the risk of **nitrosamine** formation from added nitrite, **vitamin C** is used in the curing of some brands of canned ham. See also **gammon**.

hamburger See **beefburger**.

hare A **game** mammal, with darker, richer flesh than rabbit. Hare provides **protein** and some **fat**. It is rich in well-absorbed **iron** and also contains **potassium, phosphorus** and **niacin**. It is usually served 'jugged' (stewed), in its own juices, minimizing losses of micronutrients.

haricot bean The ripe seed of a variety of French bean (a **pulse**), which is boiled and eaten as a vegetable or canned in tomato sauce (see **baked beans**). Haricot beans provide **starch, dietary fibre** and **protein**, and small amounts of **sugars** and **fat**. They have an energy value of 271 kcal/100 g (dried). Haricot beans also contain **potassium, phosphorus, iron, zinc, molybdenum** and **manga-**

nese. Like all pulses, they contain small amounts
of **phytic acid** and **lectins**, and should be thoroughly cooked to destroy these substances.

hazelnut (also called **cob nut**) The small
rounded nut of the hazel shrub, with a thin, brown
woody shell and a smooth rounded kernel. Hazelnuts are eaten whole or used whole or ground to
flavour biscuits, cakes and chocolate. They have a
high **fat** content and a correspondingly high
energy value of 380 kcal/100 g. Hazelnuts provide
dietary fibre, **protein** and some **sugars** and **starch**.
They are a rich source of **vitamin E** and a good
source of most **B complex vitamins**, except vitamin
B_{12}. Hazelnuts also contain **potassium**, **phosphorus**, **iron**, **zinc** and **manganese**.

health food A food that is considered to be
needed for a healthy diet. In general it takes in all
wholefoods, **organic foods** and dietary **supplements**. Some health foods can form part of a
healthy diet but others are less desirable. Some
make misleading claims about their beneficial
properties and others may be harmful when taken
in excess amounts. See also **megavitamin therapy**.

heart A type of **offal**, usually of a lamb or calf,
which may be served roasted or stewed. Heart
provides **protein** and variable amounts of **fat** of
which a reasonable proportion is **saturated fatty
acids**. It contains rather more **cholesterol** than
other meats and has an energy value of 119 kcal/

100 g. Heart also contains **potassium**, **phosphorus**, **iron**, **zinc**, **sulphur**, and the **B complex vitamins**. Unusually for a meat product, heart contains **vitamin C**. Some niacin, vitamin C, vitamin B_{12} and biotin may be lost when it is cooked, particularly if roasted.

heart disease Any disease affecting the functioning of the heart. The most common form of heart disease, and the one closely associated with diet, is **coronary heart disease**.

heartburn A burning sensation in the chest, caused by the regurgitation of the acidic digestive juices in the stomach, which may occur in indigestion, and may be caused or aggravated by a **hiatus hernia**. It is also a common problem in pregnancy. See also APPENDIX II, SPECIAL NEEDS.

herb tea An infusion made from any kind of herb, which may or may not have medicinal properties traditionally attributed to it. The term is also loosely applied to any kind of infusion, such as a fruit or flower infusion, that is not made from the traditional tea plant.

herb Part of an aromatic plant, usually the leaves, that is used fresh or dried, whole or ground to add flavour to food, e.g. **basil**, **oregano** and **tarragon**. Herbs have similar nutritional values to other green vegetables, but they are used in such small amounts that their contribution to nutrient intake is usually negligible.

herring A marine, soft-finned fatty fish. Herring is usually grilled or fried, and is also available pickled (see **rollmop**) or smoked (see **kipper**). It provides **protein**, a variable **fat** content and has an energy value of 199 kcal/100 g (grilled). Herring has a relatively high content of long chain essential **fatty acids** of the linolenic family. These reduce the tendency of the blood to clot and may play a part in reducing the risk of **stroke** and **heart disease**. Herring is a good source of **vitamins A**, **D** and **B₁₂** and of well-absorbed **iron** and **zinc**. It also contains **potassium**, **phosphorus**, **sulphur**, **niacin**, **biotin** and **pantothenic acid**. Some pantothenic acid is lost when it is fried.

hiatus hernia A protrusion of part of the stomach through the opening in the diaphragm where the oesophagus joins the stomach. A hiatus hernia, which most commonly occurs in those suffering from **obesity**, may be indicated by frequent **heartburn**. It can also occur in pregnancy and as a result of chronic coughing.

high blood pressure See **hypertension**.

histamine A substance released by the body tissues in many allergic reactions. In the skin this gives rise to **urticaria** or nettle rash and in the lungs to symptoms of **asthma**.

honey A sweet substance made by bees from flower nectar. It has been used as a food, preservative and a sweetener since ancient times. Honey has a high **sugars** content, of which most is fructose and glucose, and it has an energy value of 281 kcal/100 g. It contains only negligible amounts of other **nutrients** and **micronutrients**. Honey is sweeter than sucrose because of the fructose content. When honey is first made it is clear, dark and runny, but if it has not been heat treated before packaging (usually in jars), it eventually goes cloudy, pale and hard.

hormone Any of several substances secreted into the bloodstream that have specific effects upon organs and bodily processes, e.g. **insulin**. The endocrine glands, such as the **adrenal gland**, produce most of the hormones, but they are also produced by other tissues, e.g. the stomach and intestines to help the process of digestion.

hormones (in foods) Any of a variety of hormones that may be injected into livestock while they are still alive (e.g. to promote their growth and cause rapid weight gain), or after slaughter (e.g. to cause water retention in the carcass, maintaining the weight and therefore the value of the meat). These hormones may still be present in small amounts in food when it is eaten, and may cause **allergies** in some people.

horseradish The pungent white root of a Eurasian plant that is ground and made into a hot relish (usually with vinegar and seasoning).

123

Horseradish is used in such small quantities that its nutritional properties are negligible; horseradish sauce may contain additives.

hummus, hoummos or houmous A slightly grainy, off-white paste made with ground **chickpeas** and flavoured with garlic. Hummus provides the nutrients and micronutrients associated with chickpeas (**starch, protein, dietary fibre, sugars, potassium, calcium, magnesium, carotene, folic acid** and small amounts of **fat, iron** and **niacin**). It has an energy value of 185 kcal/100 g.

hydrolysed vegetable protein See **textured vegetable protein**.

hyperactivity A behavioural problem occurring in childhood, characterized by short attention span, violent outbursts and overactivity, which can cause disruption in school and at home. Controversy surrounds the role of diet in hyperactivity but some doctors recommend the elimination of all foods containing **artificial colours** (especially **tartrazine**) and **flavours**, sodium glutamate, **nitrite and nitrate**, **antioxidants**, butylated hydroxyanisole and butylated hydroxytoluene and benzoic acid. Initially foods containing natural **salicylates** are avoided.

hyperglycaemia See **blood glucose**.

hyperlipidaemia Higher than average amounts of **lipid** (**cholesterol** and **triglyceride**) in the blood.

Raised levels can be caused by a variety of factors, including diet (fat, cholesterol, carbohydrate and alcohol intakes) and genetic disorders. Raised blood cholesterol is an important risk factor in **coronary heart disease**.

hypertension High blood pressure. It is caused by genetic, environmental (stress and anxiety) and dietary factors, and is also caused by a variety of diseases, particularly of the heart and kidneys. **Obesity** is associated with hypertension and there is some evidence, though controversial, that at least in some people a high blood pressure may be the result of a high intake of **salt**. Hypertension is an important risk factor in **coronary heart disease** and **stroke**.

ice cream A sweet frozen food traditionally made with cream, egg yolks and sugar, and often flavoured with fruits. Ice cream is now more likely to contain vegetable fat, non-fat solids of milk, sugar, emulsifiers, stabilizers, flavours and colouring. Except for dairy ice cream, commercial varieties do not contain cream. About half the volume is air and half its weight is water. Ice cream provides some **protein**, **fat** and **sugars**, and has an energy value of 165 kcal/100 g. It also contains **calcium** and **potassium** but negligible amounts of other **micronutrients**.

indigestion (also called **dyspepsia**) Difficulty experienced in the digestion of food, causing pain in the abdomen, **heartburn** and **flatulence**. Indigestion may be caused by eating too quickly, or too much, by eating at times of emotional stress or by eating larger amounts than usual of fat or **dietary fibre**.

inositol A component of **phytic acid**, it is chemically an alcohol. Although often classed as a **B complex vitamin** it is not considered essential to humans. It is readily found in most diets and is also thought to be produced by the body. There is no known deficiency disease.

insecticide A chemical for killing insects. See **pesticide**.

insulin A hormone secreted by the pancreas, involved in controlling **blood glucose** levels. The release of insulin is triggered by a rise in blood sugar levels following a meal. Insulin enables body cells to take up glucose and use it immediately for energy or to store it in the form of fat, or as **glycogen** for use later. In **diabetes** there is either an insufficient or ineffective supply of insulin.

intensive farming See **factory farming**.

iodine An essential **trace element** concentrated in the thyroid gland, necessary for the production of the thyroid hormones and involved in metabolism. The best sources of iodine are **kelp** and fish but they are not eaten in sufficient amounts to make a reliable contribution to the intake. In the UK, most iodine is obtained from milk and dairy products, fish and meats. There is no UK **RDA** for iodine, but the US RDA is set at 150 µg for adults. Iodine deficiencies are localized in areas where there are low concentrations of iodine in the soil, and the population subsists on local produce only (this is rare in the UK). The deficiency causes goitre, with characteristic enlargement of the thyroid gland, and poor thyroid function. Excessive intakes of iodine are very rare.

iron A metallic **trace element** that is an important component of haemoglobin (the compound in red blood cells that transports oxygen to all parts of the body). A proportion of the body's iron is stored in the liver. The UK **RDA** for adult men is 10 mg, but women and adolescent girls have a higher RDA of 12 mg to compensate for the losses during periods. Pregnant and lactating women have an even higher RDA of 13 mg and 15 mg respectively. The best food sources of iron are black puddings, mollusc shellfish, liver, kidney, game, lentils, haricot beans, wholemeal bread and meat. The iron in animal foods is well absorbed, and absorption of iron from plant sources is improved in the presence of vitamin C. A certain amount of iron **leaches** out during cooking but can be recovered if the juices are used to make a gravy or sauce, otherwise iron contents are little affected by cooking, processing and storage. Iron deficiency causes **anaemia**. Once iron stores are full any iron excess to requirements is not absorbed but excreted in the faeces. Excess iron, usually taken in the form of supplements, can cause constipation or diarrhoea.

irradiation of food A method of food preservation that uses ionizing radiation to destroy bacteria and fungi. It does not leave the food radioactive. It can be used for four types of preservation: sterilization, pasteurization, disinfection and retardation of ripening or sprouting. Losses of **vitamin C**, **thiamin** and **vitamin E** occur when food is irradiated.

jam (also called **conserve**) A confection of sugar and fresh fruit boiled together until set. The setting power of any particular jam depends on the **pectin** content of the fruit. In jam the fruit is generally crushed or pulped during cooking, in a conserve the whole fruit is preserved in syrup. Jams have a very high sugar content and a correspondingly high energy value of 261 kcal/100 g, and they contain virtually no **micronutrients**. Low-sugar jams are also available. Manufactured jams may contain food additives, especially colourings.

jasmine tea A perfumed tea made by adding jasmine petals to Chinese **tea**. Jasmine tea is not an infusion of jasmine flowers and it does contain the **tannins** and theophylline associated with ordinary tea.

jelly A sweet, clear gel, traditionally made with fruit juice and **gelatin**, and eaten as a dessert. Commercially produced jelly, in the form of cubes or crystals to be made up with water, is made of a mixture of **sugars**, gelatin, flavour and colouring but with no fruit. Such jelly provides sugars and an energy value of 59 kcal/100 g, but insignificant amounts of other nutrients and micronutrients. Making jelly up with milk will improve the nutritional value. Homemade jelly made with fruit contains some vitamin C.

Jerusalem artichoke The smooth, pleasant tasting underground tuber of a North American variety of sunflower. Jerusalem artichokes are boiled and eaten as vegetables. They provide small amounts of inulin (a **polysaccharide**), **dietary fibre** and **protein**, and are a rich source of **potassium**. They have an energy value of 18 kcal/100 g.

joule A basic unit for measuring energy. Like the **calorie**, the joule is too small for practical use and the kilojoule (1000 joules) is used. 4.184 kilojoules are equal to 1 kilocalorie.

juice, fruit See **fruit juice**.

juice, vegetable See **vegetable juice**.

juniper berry The small purple berry of a northern hemisphere shrub, used to give flavour to foods and in the making of gin. Juniper berries are used in such small quantities in food that their nutritional properties are negligible. Infusions of the berries are traditionally used to stimulate the appetite and aid digestion.

kale A variety of cabbage with slightly bitter, dark green crinkled leaves. Kale is boiled and eaten as a vegetable. It provides some **sugars**, **dietary fibre** and **protein**, and has an energy value of 39 kcal/100 g. Kale also contains **potassium**, **manganese**, **carotene**, **vitamin C**, **folic acid** and some **iron**. Some of the vitamin C and folic acid are lost when it is boiled.

kefir A soured cows' milk made by fermenting the milk with yeast and bacteria (*Lactobacillus bulgaricus*). Kefir has a nutritional value similar to **yoghurt**.

kelp A variety of seaweed that enters the diet mostly in the form of **alginates**. Kelp is also sold as a supplement in powder or tablet form for its mineral content. It is a rich source of **iodine** and it also provides **potassium**, **calcium**, **sulphur**, **magnesium**, **iron**, **zinc**, **manganese** and **copper**. It has a high **sodium** content.

ketchup Any kind of piquant sauce made with fruits – most commonly tomatoes – vinegar and sugar. Tomato ketchup provides **sugars** and has a high **sodium** and **potassium** content, with an energy value of 98 kcal/100 g. It may contain colouring and flavouring.

ketosis A condition in which chemical groups, called ketones, are released by the incomplete metabolism of **fatty acids** in the liver. Ketosis occurs in situations where most of the energy produced by the body comes from fat rather than **carbohydrate**, e.g. in starvation, severe diabetes or a diet very rich in fat. Ketosis causes a build-up of acetone in the lungs, identifiable by the smell of acetone (similar to nail-varnish remover) on the breath.

kidney A type of **offal** from a lamb, calf, pig or ox. Kidney requires gentle cooking to avoid toughness and loss of flavour. The nutritional value of kidney varies according to the animal. In general it provides high-quality **protein** and only small amounts of **fat**, but with a high proportion of **cholesterol**, and has an energy value of approximately 90 kcal/100 g. It is a very rich source of **vitamin B$_{12}$**, a good source of well-absorbed **iron** and has a naturally high **sodium** content. Kidney also provides **potassium**, **phosphorus**, **retinol**, most other **B complex vitamins** and some **vitamin C**.

kidney bean The mature seed of several varieties of leguminous plant (**pulses**), particularly the runner and French bean, with a characteristic kidney shape and dark red skin. Kidney beans are boiled and eaten as vegetables or in salads or added to meat dishes. They provide **starch**, some **sugars** and **dietary fibre**, **protein** and very little **fat**, and have an energy value of 272 kcal/100 g (dried). Kidney beans also contain **potassium**, **calcium**, **magnesium**, **phosphorus**, **iron**, **manganese**, **molybdenum**, **folic acid** and some **niacin**. There are few losses of micronutrients in canned kidney beans. As with other pulses, they may contain **phytic acid** and **lectins**, and they should be cooked thoroughly to destroy these substances. Kidney beans are often used as a meat substitute in a vegetarian diet.

kilocalorie (kcal)   One thousand **calories**.

kilojoule (kJ)   One thousand **joules**.

kipper   A salted, smoked **herring**, usually baked or grilled. Kippers have a similar nutritional value to herring except that they are highly salted and have a very high **sodium** content.

kiwi fruit   The oval fruit of an Asian climbing plant, with thin furry skin, smooth, bright green flesh and tiny black pips. Kiwi fruits provide **sugars**, some **dietary fibre**, small amounts of **protein** and have an energy value of 54 kcal/100 g. They are a good source of **vitamin C**.

kohlrabi   The thickened, white stem of a variety of cabbage, that is boiled and eaten as a vegetable. Kohlrabi provides some **sugars**, **dietary fibre** and **protein**. It also contains **potassium** and small amounts of **vitamin C** and **iron**. Some of the vitamin C is lost when it is cooked.

kosher food   Food that is acceptable to orthodox Jews, having been prepared according to Jewish dietary laws.

kumquat   The tiny oval fruit of a small Chinese tree, similar to a miniature orange, with bright orange, sweet skin and very sour flesh. Kumquats are eaten raw, including the skin, or used to make jam and to give flavour to dishes. They contain **sugars** and **vitamin C**, and have an energy value of 138 kcal/100 g.

lactic acid   A weak acid produced when **glucose** is metabolized to release energy in the absence of oxygen. Lactic acid is used as a preservative to prevent growth of bacteria that cause food spoilage. It occurs naturally in sour milk, molasses and some fruits. Production of yoghurt, sour cream and some cheeses depends on the formation of lactic acid by bacteria as they feed on the sugars present.

lactose   A simple carbohydrate or **disaccharide** of **glucose** and **galactose** found in milk. Lactose is less sweet than **sucrose** but has the same energy value. It is broken down by the enzyme lactase in the digestive tract into its constituent monosaccharides (glucose and galactose), which are absorbed and carried in the blood to the liver and used for energy supply.

lactose intolerance   An inability to digest **lactose** caused by a lack of the enzyme lactase (which breaks down lactose into glucose and galactose) in the body. In lactose intolerance, undigested lactose is fermented in the large intestine by bacteria and **lactic acid** is produced. This causes abdominal discomfort and diarrhoea. Lactose intolerance affects older children and adults, and is common in many parts of the world. This may be a genetic characteristic, or because in these countries milk is not consumed after early childhood and so the ability to produce lactase is lost.

ladies' fingers   See **okra**.

laetrile   A chemical substance obtained from apricot stones which has been claimed to cure cancer. It is not a vitamin and has not been shown to have any effect on the body other than the possible toxic action from its cyanide content.

lager   A pale light-bodied beer. Lagers are made with yeasts that ferment at the bottom of the vat and increase the effervescence. They contain less **alcohol** than beers and stout, small amounts of **sugars** and have an energy value of 29 kcal/100 g (sixth of a pint).

lamb   The meat of a young sheep, less than one year old. The **nutrient** content of lamb is similar for all the various cuts, although shoulder and chops have more **fat**. The fat content, containing a high proportion of **saturated fatty acids**, can be reduced by trimming away any visible fat. Lamb provides **protein**, well-absorbed **iron** and **zinc**, **phosphorus** and small amounts of **thiamin**, **riboflavin** and **vitamin B$_{12}$**. See also **mutton**.

lard Rendered and clarified pig fat, especially from the abdomen, used in cooking. It contains a high proportion of **saturated fatty acids** and has a very high energy value of 891 kcal/100 g, but only negligible amounts of other **nutrients** and **micronutrients**. **Antioxidants** are permitted in lard.

laxative A substance that stimulates the evacuation of the faeces. Some natural substances have a mild laxative effect, e.g. liquorice and molasses. If laxatives are needed regularly, medical advice should be sought. If laxatives are overused (as in the case of **bulimia nervosa**) they cause diarrhoea, which dehydrates the body, reduces the absorption of nutrients and upsets the body's **acid-base balance**.

leaching The draining of vitamins and minerals from foods during cooking into the cooking water, or during thawing into the drip. The vitamins most likely to be lost by leaching are the **B complex vitamins** (especially niacin, folic acid, thiamin and riboflavin) and **vitamin C**. The losses can be minimized by using very little cooking water and not discarding the water afterwards but using it to make gravy or sauces. Some minerals, e.g. **potassium** and **magnesium**, are also leached into cooking water. Up to 66% of the magnesium can be lost when vegetables are boiled but it is recovered if the liquid is used for sauce or gravy.

lead A toxic metallic element not essential for man. Lead is present in the body in very small quantities and levels of more than 30 µg/100 ml blood indicate excessive exposure. Even higher concentrations are associated with lead poisoning, to which children are particularly susceptible. Lead is absorbed from food, water (where lead pipes are still used), cigarette smoke or from vehicle exhaust fumes, although greater use of lead-free petrol is reducing lead levels in the atmosphere. Lead is excreted from the body very slowly, so it is possible for regular intakes of lead to build up to toxic levels. Lead poisoning causes **anaemia** and damage to the kidneys and nervous system.

lecithin A **phospholipid** found in most foods. It is not an essential nutrient because it can be produced in the body. Lecithin is found in the bloodstream and in the protective sheath around nerves. It is produced commercially from soya beans and other oil seeds and is widely used in the food industry as an emulsifier.

lectins Substances found in most **pulses**, particularly raw or undercooked kidney beans, butter beans and runner beans. Lectins are toxic but they are destroyed by boiling (dried beans must be boiled for at least 10 minutes) or by **sprouting**. If lectins are ingested, they can cause nausea, vomiting and diarrhoea.

leeks Vegetables of the lily family, related to the onion, in which the elongated bulb root and leaves are eaten. Leeks contain **sugars**, some **dietary fibre** and small amounts of **protein**. They have an energy value of 24 kcal/100 g (boiled) and provide **iron** and small amounts of vitamins and minerals. The leaves are a rich source of **carotene**, but the root contains only negligible amounts.

legumes Another name for **pulses**.

lemon A small, yellow and very acidic citrus fruit native to Southeast Asia, used particularly for flavouring both sweet and savoury foods. Lemons contain **dietary fibre**, some **sugars**, only a very small amount of **protein** and have an energy value of 15 kcal/100 g. They are an excellent source of **vitamin C**. They also contain **calcium**, **copper**, **vitamin B$_6$** and **pantothenic acid**. The rind of lemons contains **pectin**.

Lemon juice has none of the **dietary fibre** and only half the **sugars** and **protein** present in a whole lemon, and an energy value of 7 kcal/100 g. Many of the micronutrients are also lost when lemons are squeezed, but the juice retains more than half the **vitamin C** content. Lemon juice is acidic and may aggravate gastric ulcers.

lemon balm tea An infusion made from the

137

leaves of the lemon balm plant. Lemon balm is traditionally used for its general soothing effect.

lemon barley water   See **barley water**.

lemon grass   A herb valued for its antiseptic qualities. Lemon grass taken as a tea is traditionally used to alleviate fevers and relieve the symptoms of colds and influenza.

lemon juice   See **lemon**.

lemon sole   See **sole**.

lemonade   A refreshing drink traditionally made with fresh lemon juice, sugar and water. It contains some **vitamin C**. Manufactured lemonade contains artificially carbonated water, sugar, citric acid and flavourings. It has an energy value of 21 kcal/100 g but no other nutritional value. Low-calorie lemonade is also available.

lentil   A highly nutritious **pulse** originating from Southwest Asia. Red, green, and brown lentils all have similar nutritional values. They are rich in **protein** and **starch**, provide **dietary fibre** and some **sugars**, and have an energy value of 304 kcal/100 g. Lentils contain **potassium**, **phosphorus**, **copper**, **sulphur**, **molybdenum**, **thiamin**, **niacin**, **vitamin B$_6$** and **pantothenic acid**. They contain **iron**, **zinc**, **calcium** and **magnesium**, but also **phytic acid**, which interferes with the absorption of these minerals.

More iron is absorbed if lentils are eaten with foods containing **vitamin C**. Many of the **micro-nutrients** are depleted by boiling, but this can be avoided if the lentils are allowed to absorb all the water by the time they are cooked. Lentils may also be **sprouted**. **Lectins** present in lentils are broken down by cooking for at least 10 minutes, and phytic acid is broken down by soaking the lentils in water.

lettuce A leafy green vegetable. Lettuce has a very high water content, provides little **dietary fibre**, **sugars** and **protein**, and has an energy value of 12 kcal/100 g. It is a valuable source of **carotene** (particularly the greener leaves), **vitamin C** and **folic acid**.

lime A small, green citrus fruit. Limes, or their juice, are usually used as a flavouring. They have a less sour flavour than **lemons**. They are very similar to lemons in nutritional value, but they contain a little more sugar and less **vitamin C**. Limes have an energy value of 36 kcal/100 g, and the rind of limes contains **pectin**.

linoleic acid An essential **fatty acid**. Linoleic acid is a **polyunsaturated fatty acid** that the body cannot synthesize and it must, therefore, be obtained from the diet. The richest natural sources are corn oil, safflower-seed oil, sesame seed oil, soya bean oil and sunflower oil.

lipids The biochemical term for fatty substances in the body. See **fat**; **fatty acids**; **polyunsaturated fatty acids**; **saturated fatty acids**.

lipoprotein A **protein** combined with a **lipid**, formed in the body to transport water-insoluble fat in the blood. **Cholesterol** and **triglycerides** are carried as lipoproteins in the body. A high level of low-density lipoproteins (LDL) is associated with an increased risk of **coronary heart disease**. Reducing total fat, particularly fats with a high proportion of **saturated fatty acids**, can lower LDL levels. A high level of high-density lipoproteins (HDL) has a protective effect against coronary heart disease. HDL is not altered by diet, but regular exercise, maintaining an acceptable body weight and giving up smoking can raise HDL levels.

liqueur An alcoholic syrup distilled from wine or brandy and flavoured with fruits or herbs. Liqueurs have a high sugar content and an energy value of 311 kcal/100 ml (three measures), but are deficient in all other **nutrients** and **micronutrients**. The **alcohol** content of liqueurs varies between 17% and 23% by volume.

liquorice An extract of the root of a Mediterranean shrub used in confectionery and as a flavouring. Traditionally liquorice has been used as a mild **laxative**, to soothe sore throats, act as an expectorant and, until recently, to treat peptic ulcers. Confectionery liquorice contains **sugars**, some **starch**, a small amount of **fat** and has an energy value of 293 kcal/100 g. It also contains high levels of **iron**. Confectionery liquorice may contain colouring, flavouring and preservatives.

listeria A type of bacteria commonly found in soil, water and the digestive system of animals. It can enter the human body through unwashed vegetables (including salad vegetables), unhygienically prepared cook-chill foods and some soft cheeses. The presence of listeria in the body does not usually cause any problems as there is an inbuilt resistance, but people with lowered immunity can contract listeriosis. Those at risk are pregnant women, babies, the elderly and the sick, particularly AIDS and cancer patients. The incubation period can last up to several weeks and the symptoms are flu-like, including high temperatures and dizziness. Listeriosis can cause miscarriages, meningitis and even death.

liver **Offal** of lamb, pig, calf, ox and poultry. The nutrient contents vary with species and age of the animal, but generally liver provides **protein**, some **fat** (saturated) and has an average energy value of 157 kcal/100 g. Liver is a good source of well-absorbed **iron**, **copper**, **zinc**, **vitamin A**, **vitamin B_{12}**, **folic acid**, **riboflavin**, **vitamin B_6** and **pantothenic acid**. It also contains smaller amounts of **vitamin C** and other vitamins and minerals. Liver paté contains more liver than liver sausage, both have higher fat contents than liver, and a correspondingly higher energy value of 310 kcal/100 g and contain added salt.

lobster A crustacean **shellfish**. Lobster provides **protein**, little **fat** and has an energy value of 119 kcal/100 g (boiled). It has a fairly high **sodium** content and also contains some **copper**, **zinc**, **sulphur**, **niacin**, **folic acid**, **pantothenic acid** and biotin. Lobster may be eaten with butter, mayonnaise or cream, which will increase the fat content and energy value.

loganberry The dark red fruit of a trailing, prickly shrub, a cross between a raspberry and a blackberry, which is more acid than the blackberry but less intensely flavoured than the raspberry. Fresh loganberries are low in **sugars** (mostly glucose and fructose) and so have a low energy value of 17 kcal/100 g. Canned loganberries contain added sugar and have a higher energy value of 101 kcal/100 g. Loganberries provide **dietary fibre** and small amounts of **protein**. They also contain **potassium**, **iron** and **carotene**. They contain more **vitamin C** than raspberries and blackberries, but some of the vitamin C is lost if they are stewed, and most of it is lost if they are canned.

lovage A European plant with a strong celery taste whose leaves are used for flavouring food.

low-calorie Having a reduced energy content. For a product to be labelled low-calorie, it must provide 40 kcal or less per 100 g, or what is deemed to be one serving, of the standard product. This is achieved by replacing **fat**, **starch** and **sugar** in the standard product with air, water or **sweeteners**. Manufacturers are bound by law to indicate on the packages of low-calorie foods that the products 'can only help weight loss as part of a calorie-controlled diet'.

low-fat spread An emulsion of oil and water used as an alternative to margarine and butter. Low-fat spreads contain half the fat of butter and margarine and have a correspondingly lower energy value of 366 kcal/100 g. They contain variable amounts of **polyunsaturated fatty acids** depending on the oil used in manufacture. Low-fat spreads are required by law to contain added **vitamin A** and **D**, and they are permitted to contain flavouring, colouring, emulsifiers and **antioxidants**.

luncheon meat A canned meat product usually made from ground pork and cereals. Luncheon meat has a minimum legal requirement for lean meat content. It provides **protein**, a high **fat** content with a high proportion of **saturated fatty acids**, some **starch** and an energy value of 313 kcal/100 g. Luncheon meat contains added salt and, therefore, has a very high **sodium** content. It also provides small amounts of **iron**, **copper**, **zinc**, **phosphorus**, **sulphur**, **niacin** and **pantothenic acid**. Luncheon meat may contain added preservatives (including **nitrite**), **monosodium glutamate** and colouring.

lychee   The small, round fruit of a Chinese tree, with dry, uneven pinkish skin and smooth, white juicy and very sweet flesh round a smooth oval stone. Lychees provide **sugars** and only very small amounts of **dietary fibre** and **protein**, and they have an energy value of 64 kcal/100 g. They also contain good amounts of **vitamin C**. Canned lychees contain more sugars and less vitamin C than the fresh fruit.

mace   A spice obtained by drying and grinding the fleshy coating of **nutmeg** seeds to an orange-brown colour. It has a more delicate flavour than nutmeg and is used in a variety of meat and fish dishes as well as in cakes and puddings. Mace is used in such small quantities that its nutritional properties are negligible.

mackerel   A fatty fish. Mackerel provides **protein**, **fat**, with a high proportion of **polyunsaturated fatty acids**, and an energy value of 223 kcal/100 g. It is a good source of well-absorbed **iron** and **vitamin A** and B_{12}. Mackerel also provides **potassium**, **selenium**, **copper**, **zinc**, **vitamin D**, **niacin**, **vitamin B_6**, **riboflavin**, **pantothenic acid** and **biotin**. Smoked mackerel has a high **sodium** content.

macrobiotics   A diet based on keeping a balance between Yin and Yang (two complementary prin-

ciples of Chinese philosophy). Yin represents
acidity (potassium, sugar, and fruits) and Yang
alkalinity (sodium, salt and cereals). Gradually,
through seven levels of diet, the proportion of
animal products, fruit and vegetables is reduced
towards the final goal of eating only brown rice
(level seven). See also APPENDIX II, VEGETARIAN,
VEGAN AND MACROBIOTIC DIETS.

macronutrient A general term for all sub-
stances, e.g. **protein**, **fat**, **carbohydrate** and **dietary
fibre**, required in the diet in larger quantites than
micronutrients.

magnesium An essential mineral that together
with calcium forms an integral part of bones and
teeth. Magnesium is also involved in energy
supply, nerve and muscle function and the utilization of calcium and potassium. Magnesium is
widespread in foods, especially those of vegetable
origin, and particularly good sources are nuts,
wholegrain cereals, green vegetables and cocoa
powder. There is no UK **RDA**, but the US RDA is
350 mg. Pregnant, lactating and menstruating
women need a higher daily intake of 450 mg. Magnesium deficiency due to inadequate diet is
unlikely because it is so widespread in food. A
number of conditions may prevent magnesium
absorption and lead to a deficiency, for example
excessive **alcohol** intake, use of **diuretics**, prolonged diarrhoea and diseases of **malabsorption**.
Magnesium deficiency initially causes general

weakness and apathy leading to convulsions and eventually death from heart attack.

maize A cereal used globally as a source of energy and for its oil. In Britain, maize is most commonly eaten as breakfast cereal or popcorn. Maize provides **starch**, little **protein** and some **fat**, but it is deficient in an essential **amino acid** and has an energy value of 353 kcal/100 g. It also contains **iron**, **phosphorus**, **manganese** and **molybdenum**, and some **thiamin** and **riboflavin**. See also **cornflour**; **sweetcorn**.

maize oil See **corn oil**.

malabsorption A failure in the ability to absorb one or more **nutrients**. There are many possible causes, including enzyme deficiency, infection, a reduction in the intestinal surface for absorption because of surgery and insufficient bile production for fat absorption. Features of malabsorption syndrome include diarrhoea, abdominal distension, flatulence and, with time, weight loss and nutritional deficiencies such as **anaemia**, electrolyte and fluid loss and **osteomalacia**.

malic acid A harmless acidic substance present in some fruits. The greatest quantities of malic acid are found in apples, and in tomatoes and plums. It has a distinctively fruity flavour and is sometimes used as a flavouring by manufacturers.

malnutrition A lack or excess of one, or more often, several **nutrients** in the diet. This may result from starvation, **malabsorption** or from a badly balanced diet (see the introductory chapter, A BALANCED DIET).

malt extract A syrup derived from malted barley and traditionally used to flavour **cod-liver oil** supplements. Malt extract is now used as a flavouring in many kinds of biscuit and bread. It has a high **sugars** content and an energy value of 304 kcal/100 g, but negligible amounts of **nutrients** and **micronutrients**.

maltose A simple carbohydrate or **disaccharide** of two **glucose** units. Maltose is less sweet than **sucrose** but has the same energy value of 394 kcal/100 g. It is produced when **starch** is broken down by enzymes in the digestive tract. Further enzymatic action reduces maltose to its constituent monosaccharide glucose, which is then absorbed and carried in the blood to the liver and used for energy supply. Maltose occurs naturally in small amounts, particularly in honey and sprouted wheat and barley.

mandarin (also called **mandarin orange**) A small orange-like citrus fruit with a characteristic loose skin. Mandarins provide **sugars**, little **protein** and **dietary fibre** and have an energy value of 25 kcal/100 g. They also contain reliable amounts of **vitamin C** and small amounts of **carotene** and **folic acid**. Mandarins canned in syrup have a higher sugars content and an energy value of 57 kcal/100 g and those canned in natural juice have an energy value of 39 kcal/100 g. About half the vitamin C content is lost when mandarins are canned.

manganese A **trace element** that is a component of many enzyme systems and is important in reproduction. Manganese is found in nuts, wholegrain cereals, pulses, leafy green vegetables and fruit; tea is very rich in manganese. There is no UK **RDA**, but a daily intake of 2.5–5 mg is considered adequate. No disease syndrome is associated with a deficiency of manganese.

mangetout (also called **sugar pea**) The immature pod of the garden pea. Mangetout provides only small amounts of **protein**, **sugars**, **starch** and **dietary fibre**, and has an energy value of 43 kcal/100 g (boiled). Mangetout are **pulses**, but because they are eaten in the immature state, their nutritional value closely resembles that of the runner bean. If mangetout are to be used in a salad, they should be **parboiled** first to ensure the breakdown of **lectins** that may be present.

mango The sweet, fragrant fruit of the tropical mango tree. Mangoes have a high **sugars** content, provide only small amounts of **protein** and **dietary fibre**, and have an energy value of 59 kcal/100 g. Ripe mangoes are high in **carotene** and **vitamin C**. Mangoes canned in syrup have a higher sugars content and a correspondingly higher energy value of 77 kcal/100 g. Much of the vitamin C content is lost when mangoes are canned.

maple syrup   A fragrant syrup extracted from the sap of the sugar maple tree. Maple syrup has a very high **sugars** content and an energy value of 250 kcal/100 g but negligible amounts of other **nutrients** and **micronutrients**.

margarine   A spread made from vegetable or animal oils. Margarines can be hard or soft and used for spreading like butter or for cooking. They are almost 100% **fat**. The type of oil used and the method of manufacture determine the proportions of **fatty acids** in the finished product. Some contain a high proportion of polyunsaturated fatty acids and will be labelled as such, others may have a high proportion of saturated fatty acids. All types of margarine have an energy value of 730 kcal/100 g and are a good source of **vitamin E**. **Vitamins A** and **D** are added by law to all margarines and those containing added salt have high **sodium** contents. Margarines may contain flavouring, colouring, emulsifiers and **antioxidants**.

marjoram (also called **sweet marjoram**)   The leaves of a small Mediterranean plant used fresh or dried, whole or powdered, as a herb. Marjoram is consumed in such small quantities that its nutritional value is negligible.

marrow   The large edible fruit of a creeping plant. Marrows are eaten as vegetables or sometimes used in chutney and jam. They have a high water content, contain only small amounts of **sugars**, **dietary fibre**, and **protein**, and have an energy value of 7 kcal/100 g (boiled). Marrows contain negligible amounts of micronutrients.

meat   The edible flesh of animals, such as **beef**, **game**, **lamb**, **mutton**, **pork** and **veal**, including sinews, gristle and **offal**, as well as flesh from the head, **tongue**, neck and tail. The nutritional content and energy value of meat varies enormously according to the animal and the part of the body it comes from, and the amount of **fat** included. In general, it provides **protein** and varying amounts of fat with a high proportion of **saturated fatty acids**. Meat contains well-absorbed **iron** and **zinc** as well as useful amounts of **phosphorus**, **niacin**, **riboflavin**, **thiamin** and **vitamin B$_{12}$**.

The fat content of meat is both visible and invisible (i.e. the fat that is part of the muscle). Lean meat has the visible fat removed and the invisible fat reduced by breeding methods; it has a maximum fat content of 10%. The fattiest cuts of meat, e.g. breast of lamb, contain 35% fat. The white meat from **poultry** has a relatively low fat content, and most of it is in the skin and so easily removed. The fat levels can be further reduced by grilling rather than frying. For ways of lowering the amount of fat in the diet see the introductory chapter A BALANCED DIET.

It is necessary to cook meat to destroy any harmful bacteria and to make the muscle fibres more digestible. However, nutrient loss occurs in some cooking methods, and to restore some of the nutrients **leached** during cooking a sauce or gravy should be made from the juices. The vitamin B_{12} content of meat is reduced when it is boiled, braised or stewed, but losses are less when grilled or roasted. When frozen meat is thawed **pantothenic acid** and other **B complex vitamins** are lost in the drip. See **bacon**; **beefburger**; **cured meats**; **gammon**; **ham**; **kidney**; **luncheon meat**; **mince**; **paté**; **sausage**; **steak**; **stewing steak**. See also **hormones (in food)**.

meat substitute   See **novel protein food**.

megavitamin therapy   The taking of very large doses – usually more than 10 times the **RDA** – of vitamins based on the incorrect theory that very large doses of vitamins confer special benefits. Megavitamin therapy is a controversial form of therapy, used more widely in the US than in the UK. The few properly conducted trials that have been carried out have failed to show any convincing benefits other than those due to the placebo effect. Regular megadosing with vitamins can lead to accumulation of toxic levels of fat-soluble vitamins (**vitamins A**, **D**, **E** and **K**) in the body. Large doses of even the water-soluble vitamins (**B complex vitamins** and **vitamin C**) may not be without danger.

melon   The edible fruits of several different twining plants with different skin and flesh colours. The most common varieties are canteloupe, honeydew and watermelon. Melons have a very high water content, provide some **sugars**, very small amounts of **protein** and **dietary fibre**, and have an energy value of 21 kcal/100 g. They also contain some **potassium**, **sulphur**, **carotene** (canteloupe melons provide much more carotene than honeydew melons), **vitamin C**, **folic acid** and **pantothenic acid**.

metabolism The combination of all the chemical processes that take place within the body. These metabolic processes include the breaking down of food into **proteins**, **carbohydrates** and **fats**; their further breakdown into **amino acids**, **monosaccharides** and **fatty acids**; their utilization for energy release and energy storage.

micronutrient A general term for all the **vitamins**, **minerals** and **trace elements** that are needed in the diet in much smaller amounts than the **macronutrients**.

microwave cooking A method of cooking in which food is heated by the vibration of the individual molecules (particularly water molecules) within the food. The vibration is caused by powerful electromagnetic radiation. Microwave cooking retains at least as much of the **micronutrient** content as conventional cooking. Because no fat is added in cooking, it can help in cutting down fat consumption. Reheating food in a microwave cooker should be as good as or superior to conventional forms of heating for conserving nutrients.

migraine A severe recurrent throbbing headache caused by constriction and subsequent dilation of blood vessels. The onset of a migraine may be indicated by partial loss of vision, and the migraine itself may be accompanied by nausea or even vomiting. Migraines are believed to be triggered by stress, hormonal factors and diet. The common dietary causes of migraine include chocolate, alcoholic drinks, cheese and citrus fruits and the food additives **tartrazine** and benzoic acid. Migraine sufferers may be able to isolate and therefore avoid those foods which cause an attack.

milk The nutritious liquid produced and secreted by the mammary glands of female mammals to feed their young. Milk differs in nutritional composition according to the species and a young mammal is best fed on the milk of its own species. Human breast milk is best for human babies and cows' milk must be modified to make it a suitable alternative to breast milk (see APPENDIX II, SPECIAL NEEDS).

The milk most commonly consumed by the UK population is cows' milk. **Ewes' milk**, **goats' milk** and **soya milk** may be tolerated by those allergic to cows' milk, and soya milk is also a suitable alternative to cows' milk for **vegans**. Whole cows' milk contains 3.9 g/100 ml fat, semi-skimmed 1.7 and skimmed 0.1 g/100 ml. Milk fat contains a high proportion of **saturated fatty acids**. Milk provides **protein** and is an important source of **calcium**. It also provides some **zinc**, **potassium** and **phosphorus**. Semi-skimmed and skimmed milk do not contain any **vitamin A**, **D** and **E** because these are removed when the fat is skimmed off, but whole milk does contain these vitamins. Whole, semi-skimmed and skimmed milk are all good sources of **riboflavin** and also contain **thiamin**, **pyridoxine**, **niacin**, **folic acid**, **vitamin B$_{12}$** and **biotin**. The riboflavin content is easily destroyed by the action of sunlight, and to preserve it milk should not be left outside for any length of time. Some milks are fortified with calcium and vitamin D, but this must be clearly declared on the label. The energy values of whole, semi-skimmed and skimmed milk are 68 kcal, 48 kcal and 34 kcal/100 ml.

Most milk undergoes some form of heat treatment to destroy bacteria and improve the keeping qualities. Such treatments, **pasteurization**, **ultra heat treatment**, sterilization, evaporation, condensation and drying all cause some micronutrient loss, of which evaporation is the most destructive. As the water content is reduced in condensed, evaporated and dried milk so the energy value and nutrient content is increased, but on reconstitution with water these milks assume energy values and nutrient contents similar to the original whole, semi-skimmed or skimmed milk. Unpasteurized milk that has not been treated in any way can only be sold if the milk has come from specially accredited herds.

millet A cereal similar in nutritional composition to **wheat**. It contains **protein** and **starch**, and has an energy value of 354 kcal/100 g. Millet does not contain **gluten** and is therefore not suitable for making leavened bread.

mince Ground meat, most commonly of **beef**. Minced beef provides **protein**, variable amounts of **fat** with a high proportion of **saturated fatty acids**, so has a correspondingly variable energy value. Lean minced beef provides a maximum fat content of 10% and an energy value of 196 kcal/100 g. All minced beef contains well-absorbed **iron** and **zinc**, and all the other **micronutrients** found in beef. Mince from other animals will have a nutritional and energy value similar to the meat from which it is made. See **lamb**; **pork**; **veal**.

mineral hydrocarbons Substances derived from mineral oils such as paraffin. They are permitted for use as food additives in six foods: dried fruit, to keep the fruit moist; citrus fruit, as a coating for the skin; sweets, as a polish or glazing agent; chewing gum, as an ingredient; eggs and cheese, as a preservative coating. The use of mineral hydrocarbons is currently under review. They are considered to interfere with the absorption of nutrients, and it is likely that they will be banned from use in foods.

mineral water Water that contains dissolved minerals. The variety and concentration of the minerals depends on the source of the water, but by law there can be no more than a total of 2 g/litre of minerals. **Calcium**, **magnesium**, **potassium**, **bicarbonate** and **sulphate** are the most common minerals present. Mineral waters may be still or carbonated, naturally or artificially. Some mineral waters have a naturally high **sodium** content. Mineral waters are not treated with **chloride** or **fluoride**, their **pH** level is not altered and they do not contain toxic lead, which tap water can pick up from pipes. Mineral waters are drunk for their taste and purity, but the extra minerals taken in are negligible compared with the dietary intake as a whole.

minerals Metallic or non-metallic elements that are essential to the body and must be provided by the diet. Their main functions are as components of bones and teeth, regulators of the composition of body fluids and as necessary substances for the correct functioning of many **enzymes**. **Calcium**, **chloride**, **magnesium**, **phosphorus**, **potassium**, **sodium** and **sulphur** are required in amounts greater than 100 mg per day. The **trace elements**, **chromium**, **cobalt**, **copper**, **fluoride**, **iodine**, **iron**, **manganese**, **molybdenum**, **selenium** and **zinc**, are needed in amounts less than 100 mg or even less than 1 mg per day. Other minerals are present in the body and may be essential, but their functions are not yet clearly understood. These minerals are arsenic, **nickel**, **silicon**, **tin** and vanadium. Some elements may be present in the body but are known to be toxic; these include **cadmium**, **lead** and **mercury**. An **RDA** (recommended daily amount) for some minerals has been established to act as a guideline to requirements. However, this figure varies according to age, sex and occupation, and may be affected by illness, pregnancy, lactation and times of stress or rigorous activity. A deficiency in any mineral should be corrected by increasing consumption of foods that are rich in that mineral. A mineral supplement may be needed in some cases. For the individual functions, food sources, RDA and deficiency symptoms of the minerals, see the individual entries.

mint A plant whose aromatic leaves are used fresh or dried, whole or powdered, as a herb. Mint is consumed in such small quantities that its nutritional value is negligible. It contains menthol and **tannins** and the leaves are used to make a refreshing infusion. See also **peppermint tea**.

modified starch A form of **starch** that has been treated with heat, enzymes or chemicals so that it maintains its consistency when it is used by manufacturers to thicken and bind foods. At present the use of modified starches is not controlled by law, but it is likely that they will be soon, and as food **additives** many will be allocated E numbers.

molasses A dark, thick and slightly bitter syrup obtained during the refining of cane or beet sugar.

It is a very rich source of **iron** and **calcium** and it also provides **copper**, **magnesium**, **potassium** and **zinc**. Molasses is high in **sugar** and has a high energy value of 278 kcal/100 g. It has a mild **laxative** effect.

molybdenum A **trace element** possibly essential for humans. It is a component of several important **enzymes**. It contributes to the excretion of uric acid from the body, to the utilization of iron and to the metabolism of fats. Molybdenum acts with **fluoride** in protecting tooth enamel from **dental caries**. It occurs naturally in most forms of plant life, but concentrations vary according to the soil in which the plants are grown. Good sources are wholegrain cereals, pulses, leafy vegetables, wheatgerm and liver. Some molybdenum is lost during refining processes. There is no UK or USA **RDA** for molybdenum and no deficiency disease has been linked with inadequate intake. Rare excesses of molybdenum are associated with an increased susceptibility to **gout**.

monkey nut Another name for **peanut**.

monosaccharide One of a group of simple **carbohydrates** or **sugars**, including **glucose**, **galactose**, and **fructose**. They occur in nature but only in small amounts. Monosaccharides are much more commonly found linked together as **disaccharides** and **polysaccharides**. They are the final breakdown products of carbohydrate in the digestive tract and are absorbed and carried in the blood to the liver and used for energy supply.

monosodium glutamate (MSG) A flavour enhancer made from wheat **gluten**, and used as a food additive in a wide range of savoury foods. It is not permitted in baby foods. As the sodium salt of the **amino acid** glutamic acid it has a high **sodium** content. If consumed in large amounts it may provoke a number of unpleasant effects for some people, such as a burning sensation across the back of the neck, tightness in the chest, sweating and headaches. These symptoms are described as the **Chinese restaurant syndrome**, because of the wide use of monosodium glutamate in Chinese cooking.

mooli See **radish**.

mould Microscopic fungi that may be present in certain foods and may grow and spread, especially in warm, damp conditions, causing food spoilage. Moulds not only damage food and impair its flavour, they may release toxins such as **aflatoxins** and mycotoxins. It is essential to avoid all mouldy food as many of the toxic substances are suspected carcinogens. Trimming mould off the surface is not enough as the toxins migrate into the food. All mouldy food should be thrown away.

MSG See **monosodium glutamate**.

muesli A breakfast cereal. Traditionally, muesli is a mixture of cereals, nuts and dried fruit. It may also contain seeds and bran and may be sweetened with sugar or honey. In general, mueslis provide **protein, dietary fibre, calcium, iron, thiamin, riboflavin** and **niacin**. The energy value depends on the ingredients used and can vary between 250 and 450 kcal/100 g.

muesli bar A snack bar made with cereals, seeds, vegetable oil, nuts and dried fruit and sweetened with sugars and syrups. The nutritional and energy value varies according to the ingredients.

mullet Small white fish of two distinct varieties: red mullet and grey mullet. Both varieties provide **protein**, are low in **fat** and have energy values of approximately 150 kcal/100 g. They contain small amounts of **potassium, niacin, vitamin E, vitamin B_6, vitamin B_{12}, folic acid** and **biotin**. The liver of red mullet is often cooked in the fish and if eaten increases the vitamin content.

mung bean A small, dark green **pulse**. Mung beans are a good source of **protein** and also provide **starch, dietary fibre**, small amounts of **sugars**, and little **fat**. They have an energy value of 231 kcal/100 g. They provide **potassium, calcium, magnesium, iron, copper** and **folic acid**, and small amounts of **manganese, molybdenum, thiamin, riboflavin, niacin** and **vitamin B_6**. They can either be cooked (in which case much of the thiamin is lost and the mineral content is reduced) or soaked until they sprout. Any **phytic acid** and **lectins** present in mung beans are broken down when the beans are cooked or sprouted.

mushroom Edible fungus of many kinds, the commonest being the field mushroom. Mushrooms have a high water content, contain little **protein**, a small amount of **dietary fibre** and have an energy value of 13 kcal/100 g. They are rich in **niacin**, **riboflavin** and **pantothenic acid**, but are eaten in such small amounts that their nutritional contribution to the diet as a whole is small. Mushrooms canned in saline have a high **sodium** content.

mussel A mollusc **shellfish**. Mussels provide **protein**, little **fat** and have an energy value of 87 kcal/100 g. They contain well-absorbed **iron** and **zinc** as well as **calcium**, **copper**, **zinc**, **sulphur** and small amounts of **vitamin E**. They have a fairly high **sodium** content.

mustard A hot condiment made with the powdered seeds of the mustard plant, which contain a powerful volatile oil that gives mustard its hot taste. Mustard may be mixed simply with water or with wine, cider, beer or vinegar. It may or may not contain oil, whole mustard seeds, salt, pepper, sugar, finely chopped herbs or other flavourings. Mustard is consumed in such small quantities that its nutritional properties are negligible.

mustard and cress Young sprouts of a variety of mustard plant and garden cress. Mustard and cress stems and leaves are served in salads or used as a garnish. They have a high water content and a low energy value of 10 kcal/100 g. They provide only small amounts of **protein** and **sugars**, and contain good amounts of **vitamin C**, **dietary fibre** and **potassium**.

mutton   The meat of a mature sheep. Mutton has a similar nutritional and energy value to that of **lamb**, but the **protein** quality is lower because it contains more connective tissue and therefore more **gelatin**. Mutton is tougher than lamb and stewing is the traditional method of cooking as this tenderizes the meat.

nail   The horny proteinous plate covering the end of the fingers and toes. Although the texture and colouring of nails is often affected by a specific vitamin or mineral deficiency (e.g. the spoon-shaped nails characteristic of iron-deficiency anaemia) this may not be the only cause. A medical diagnosis should be sought before starting any vitamin or mineral therapy.

nectarine   A soft, sweet and juicy fruit which is a variety of **peach**. Nectarines have the colour and flavour of a peach but the texture and smooth skin of a plum. They have a nutritional composition similar to peaches, providing **sugars**, some **dietary fibre** and very little **protein**. They also contain some **carotene** and **folic acid** and have an energy value of 50 kcal/100 g.

nettle A tall, leafy weed with characteristic stinging hairs on its stem and leaves. Nettles are eaten as vegetables, in soups, salads and infusions. The sting of the stem and leaves is lost a few hours after nettles are cut or once they are cooked. Nettles have a high water content and they provide **dietary fibre**, some **sugars**, and very small amounts of **protein**. Like all dark green leafy vegetables, nettles are a good source of **folic acid**, **riboflavin**, **carotene** and **vitamin C**, although boiling will reduce the content of all but carotene.

niacin (also called **nicotinic acid**, **nicotinamide** or **niacinamide**) A **B complex vitamin**. Niacin and its derivative niacinamide play vital parts in the metabolic reactions of the body, particularly in the release of energy within the cells. Niacin can be synthesized by the body from the essential **amino acid** tryptophan, if the diet contains sufficient tryptophan, **vitamin B$_6$**, **B$_1$** and **B$_2$**. Good food sources of niacin include liver, peanuts and yeast extracts as well as meat, fish, cheese, pulses, eggs, milk, bread and coffee. Niacin is stable to heat but some is lost through **leaching** out into the cooking water or juices. The niacin in wholegrain cereals is in a bound form, which is not available unless treated with alkalis, such as in soda bread. Niacin is added by law to white bread in the UK. The UK **RDA** for niacin is 18 mg for men and 15 mg for women.

Deficiency in the UK is extremely rare and usually only occurs as a result of an underlying disease such as **malabsorption** or alcoholism. The characteristic deficiency disease of niacin is **pellagra**. Niacin is harmless when taken in excess, as it is filtered out of the bloodstream by the kidneys and dietary supplements are unnecessary in balanced diets (see the introductory chapter, A BALANCED DIET). Niacin taken in large pharmacological doses of 3 g per day (more than could be obtained from food) may help to lower blood **cholesterol**, but such treatment must be under medical supervision.

niacinamide See **niacin**.

nickel A mineral known to be an essential **trace element** for some animals and probably for humans, but its function in people is not yet understood.

nicotinamide or **nicotinic acid** See **niacin**.

nitrate and **nitrite** Substances permitted as preservatives, used in some cheeses and cured and pickled meats. They are assigned the E numbers E249, E250, E251 and E252. Nitrates occur naturally in the soil and water, and through the use of chemical fertilizers. They can be made in the body and coverted into nitrites. The low acid content of babies' stomachs makes them particularly susceptible to nitrites, and this can lead to a potentially fatal condition. Infant foods are not allowed to contain nitrites and nitrates, and families living in regions with a high nitrate content in the tap water are supplied with special water for babies. Nitrites and nitrates are used as preservatives because they are particularly effective in preventing **botulism**. Nitrites can produce minute amounts of **nitrosamines** in the body that are potentially carcinogenic, but the risks are considered small and are far outweighed by the beneficial effects of preventing botulism.

nitrosamine One of a group of substances formed by the combination of **nitrate** with compounds present in the food called amines. Nitrosamines are known to cause cancer in animals, but only when fed nitrosamines in much greater amounts than those present in meat products. Nitrates are an additive necessary to prevent multiplication of the bacteria responsible for **botulism**, which usually proves fatal. **Vitamins C** and **E** are able to inhibit the formation of some nitrosamines, at least when taken with food.

novel protein food Any form of artificial meat, e.g. **textured vegetable protein**, usually obtained by processing **soya beans** or other plant sources of protein.

nutmeg The hard, aromatic seed of an evergreen tree, used as a spice when finely grated. It is used in such small quantities that its nutritional value is negligible.

nutrient Components of food that provide the body with fuel for energy, material for growth,

repair and maintenance, and essential substances
needed to regulate these processes. The nutrients
in food are **carbohydrate**, **fat**, **protein**, **minerals** and
vitamins. Water and oxygen, although essential
for life, are not considered as nutrients, nor is
alcohol, which supplies energy but is actually
classed as a drug. See also **macronutrient**; **micronutrient**.

nutrition   The process by which the body obtains
all the nutrients from the diet, by **digestion**,
absorption and **assimilation**, and the study of that
process.

nuts   The edible kernels of the hard, woody fruit
of certain trees. Nuts are rich sources of **fat**, **protein** and **dietary fibre**, and have high energy values.
They contain **calcium**, **zinc**, **magnesium** and **iron**,
but also **phytic acid**, which makes most of these
minerals unavailable to the body. Nuts are rich in
potassium, which is well-absorbed. Unless salt is
added during roasting they are low in **sodium**. The
peanut (also called ground nut and monkey nut) is
not, in fact, a true nut but a **pulse**. See **almond**;
Brazil nut; **cashew nut**; **chestnut**; **cob nut**; **hazel nut**;
pecan nut; **pistachio nut**; **walnut**.

oatcake   A non-sweet biscuit made from oats.
Oatcakes are high in **starch**; they also contain **protein**, **fats** and **dietary fibre**, and have an energy
value of 441 kcal/100 g. They are good sources of
potassium, **magnesium**, **iron**, **copper**, **zinc** and

biotin, and contain small amounts of **thiamin**, **niacin** and **vitamin E**. They may contain added salt, sugar and other food additives.

oats A cereal used chiefly for making porridge or as the main ingredient of **muesli**. Milling removes the husk, but usually leaves the germ. Oats are high in **starch** and have a correspondingly high energy value of 401 kcal/100 g. Their **fat** content is higher than most cereals, that is why oatmeal becomes rancid so easily. Rolled oats are made by crushing the grain between heated rollers so that it is partially cooked and the enzymes that speed up rancidity are destroyed. They also contain **protein, B complex vitamins** and minerals, but like other cereals are deficient in vitamins A, C and B_{12}. Oats have been found to lower blood **cholesterol** levels; this ability has been attributed to the presence of soluble **dietary fibre**, but it may equally be due to the presence of a high proportion of **polyunsaturated fatty acids**.

obesity A condition in which an individual accumulates an excessive amount of body fat. The body of an average adult man contains about 12% of fat and that of a woman about 25%. A fat content of more than 20% in men and 30% in women is considered obese. The assessment of obesity is more usually done by determining the **body weight** and comparing it with the acceptable weight for sex, height and age.

Fat accumulates in the body when **calorie** input exceeds calorie output. There are several diseases associated with obesity, including **diabetes**, **hypertension**, **heart disease**, **osteoarthritis** and varicose veins. For ways of dealing with obesity, see APPENDIX I, LOSING AND GAINING WEIGHT.

octopus   A soft-bodied, mollusc (see **shellfish**) with eight tentacled legs. Octopus is usually eaten fried, stewed or pickled. It provides **protein**, very little **fat** and has an energy value of 68 kcal/100 g. The flesh contains a little **iron** and **vitamin A**, but few reliable analyses are available.

oedema (also called **water retention**)   The formation of an excessive amount of fluid in the body tissues. It is characterized by swelling of limbs or accumulation of fluid in the abdomen. It is associated with some heart, liver and kidney disorders and is also a common symptom of premenstrual tension. In some kidney and heart disorders, there is an excessive amount of **salt** in the tissue fluid and therefore an increase in the water that goes with it. Restricting salt intake is part of the treatment of such disorders.

offal   A general name to include everything that is removed when dressing the meat carcase, leaving only the muscle and bone. The word was originally off-fall. It now refers to the tail, **heart**, **liver**, spleen, pancreas, thymus, **tripe**, **kidneys**, **brain** and **tongue**. The nutritional content and energy value of offal depends on the organ and the animal, but in general, offal has a low fat content, provides

protein and is a particularly good source of **iron** and some vitamins.

oil of cloves The volatile oil extracted from **cloves**. It is traditionally applied direct to the gum to alleviate toothache.

oil of evening primrose See **evening primrose oil**.

oils Liquid edible fats. See also **essential oils**.

okra (also called **ladies' fingers**) The long, tapering green seed-pod of a tropical Asian and African plant, with fleshy skin and many tiny seeds in a sticky juice. Okra may be added to soups and stews or **braised** and eaten as a vegetable. It provides small amounts of **dietary fibre**, **sugars** and **protein**, and has a low energy value at 17 kcal/100 g. It contains **iron**, **carotene**, **vitamin C** and **folic acid**. Some of the vitamin C and folic acid content is lost when it is cooked, but losses are reduced if the cooking water is used.

olive The oily green or black fruit of a Mediterranean tree. Olives are unusual fruits in that they have a high **fat** content and a correspondingly high energy value of 103 kcal/100 g. They also contain some **dietary fibre** and very small amounts of **protein**, but unusually for a fruit, no sugars. They provide small amounts of **iron**, **copper** and **carotene**, with more carotene in green than black olives. They contain virtually no vitamin C or B complex vitamins. Olives may be canned or sealed in brine, and this gives them a high **sodium** content.

Olive oil contains a high proportion of **unsaturated fatty acids**, is a reasonable source of the essential fatty acid **linoleic acid** and has a very high energy value of 899 kcal/100 g.

olive oil See **olive**.

onion A pungent bulb used for flavouring and as a vegetable. Onions have a high water content, and they provide some **sugars**, small amounts of **dietary fibre** and very little **protein**. They have an energy value of 23 kcal/100 g. They also contain a little **calcium** and **folic acid**. Spring onions contain rather more nutrients than mature onions. Onions have been shown to reduce the tendency of blood to clot and this may be beneficial in protecting against heart disease and strokes.

orange A citrus fruit, with three main varieties, the smooth-skinned, sweet Valencia, the thicker-skinned navel and the bitter Seville (used for making marmalade). Oranges provide **sugars**, some **dietary fibre** and very small amounts of **protein**, and have an energy value of 35 kcal/100 g. They are a good source of **vitamin C** and also contain **folic acid**. Orange peel contains **pectin** and it may also have been treated with preservative to stop mould growth. If oranges are to be used in cooking, or for making marmalade, they should be washed first.

Orange juice provides sugars, negligible amounts of protein and has an energy value of 33 kcal/100 g. If consumed immediately after preparation the vitamin C and folic acid contents are similar to that of the whole orange. Canned orange juice retains most of its vitamin C, but it loses some of the folic acid content. Canned orange juice may be sweetened, in which case it has a higher energy value of 51 kcal/100 g. The vitamin C content of **UHT** long-life orange juice is slightly less than that of fresh, and will decline on storage and once the container is opened. Frozen orange juice retains its vitamin C content well.

orange juice   See **orange**.

oregano   The pungent leaves of a Mediterranean variety of **marjoram**, which are dried and used chopped or powdered as a herb. Oregano is used in such small quantities that its nutritional properties are negligible.

organic foods   Foods grown under the principles of organic farming, without the use of chemical fertilizers or pesticides only fertilizers derived from animals and plants. The term is often extended to include animals reared without antibiotics or hormones, or foods prepared with the minimum of processing and without the use of food additives.

osteoarthritis A disease of the joints in which the cartilage in the joints breaks down and is replaced by bone-like growths causing pain and stiffness. It is an uncomfortable condition but it does not affect the sufferer's general health. It may be aggravated by obesity, especially in the weight-bearing joints, such as the ankles, knees and hips. See also **arthritis**.

osteomalacia A disease in which there is softening of the bones. The adult equivalent to **rickets** in children, it is caused by a **vitamin D** deficiency, and may be aggravated by a **calcium** deficiency or by an inability to absorb **phosphorus**.

osteoporosis A disease in which the bones become porous and more liable to break. As the body gets older, the bones naturally become more porous; osteoporosis exaggerates this process and makes the bones painful and dangerously brittle. It usually affects the vertebral column, the thigh bone (femur) and one of the bones of the forearm (radius). Women are particularly vulnerable to osteoporosis because of hormonal changes at the menopause or after hysterectomy. Synthetic hormones slow down the loss of bone but do not prevent it. It may also be induced by prolonged immobility. The risk of developing osteoporosis can be minimized with regular exercise and a high intake of **vitamin D**, **calcium**, **fluoride** and **phosphorus** throughout life.

overweight A condition in which an individual accumulates an excessive amount of body fat. The body of an average adult man contains about 12% fat and that of a woman about 25% fat. A fat content above these levels but below 20% in men and 30% in women would be considered overweight. Fat levels greater than those would indicate the condition of **obesity**. The assessment of overweight is more usually done by determining the body weight and comparing it with the acceptable weight for sex, height and age. Fat accumulates in the body when **calorie** input exceeds calorie output. See also APPENDIX I, LOSING AND GAINING WEIGHT.

oxalic acid A naturally occurring acid that combines with calcium and magnesium during digestion and prevents these minerals being absorbed. The most concentrated sources are tea, chocolate and other cocoa products. It is also found in spinach, rhubarb and beetroot, and smaller amounts are found in beans and cereals.

oysters A mollusc **shellfish** usually eaten raw. Oysters provide **protein** and only very small amounts of **fat**. They are a very rich source of **zinc** and some types contain **vitamin C**. Oysters contain useful amounts of **iron**, **copper**, **vitamin A**, **vitamin B$_{12}$** and **biotin**, and smaller amounts of **niacin** and **folic acid**. They have a high **sodium** content.

PABA See **para-aminobenzoic acid**.

palm oil An orange-coloured oil with a distinctive flavour, extracted from the fruit of the African palm tree. The fruit is made up of a skin surrounding a fibrous pulp within which is the seed. The oil from the pulp is orange and that from the kernel is pale yellow. Palm oil is virtually 100% **fat** and has a very high energy value of 899 kcal/100 g. It is one of only two vegetable oils that contain **saturated fatty acids** (the other being coconut oil). It is a good source of **vitamin E**. Palm oil made from pulp is rich in **carotene**.

pangamic acid (also called **vitamin B₁₅**) A substance found in most foods, it is incorrectly classed as a vitamin because it possesses none of the characteristics that make it essential for growth and health. It has been suggested that it is of value in the treatment of cardiovascular and rheumatic diseases, but its effectiveness has not been proven.

pantothenic acid (also called **vitamin B₅**) A B **complex vitamin** that is part of coenzyme A, a substance involved in several metabolic functions, including energy production. Pantothenic acid is present in all food except for fats, oils and sugar. The richest sources are royal jelly, fish roe, wheat bran, wheat germ, liver, kidney, brewer's yeast, nuts and pulses. There is no UK **RDA**, but the US RDA is 10 mg, which is contained in the average UK daily diet. It occurs in greatest concentrations in unrefined foods about half is lost when wheat is milled to white flour. Pantothenic acid **leaches** out into cooking water, and like other B complex vitamins is sensitive to heat, acids and alkalis. Up to a third is lost when meat and vegetables are cooked. Freezing does not destroy the vitamin but up to a third may be lost during thawing. There can be losses of up to three-quarters from food when canned. A deficiency of pantothenic acid can occur as part of a severe general nutritional deficiency, but other causes are unknown. Lack of the vitamin in some animals causes grey hair but pantothenic acid is ineffective in preventing greying of human hair. Pantothenic acid is well tolerated in man and a dose which is unsafe has not yet been defined.

papaya (also called **pawpaw**) A pear-shaped tropical fruit with smooth orange flesh and shiny black pips. Papayas provide **sugars**, minimal amounts of **dietary fibre** and **protein**, and have an energy value of 45 kcal/100 g. They are good sources of **carotene** and **vitamin C**, and contain smaller amounts of **iron**, **copper** and **pantothenic acid**. Canned papayas usually contain added sugar and have a higher energy value of 65 kcal/100 g. Papaya contains an enzyme called papain, which breaks down proteins and is sometimes used to tenderize meat.

para-aminobenzoic acid (also called **PABA**) A component of the vitamin **folic acid**, it is not, itself, a vitamin. Although essential for some organisms, it is not for humans who depend on a

175

dietary supply of folic acid. PABA is used as a sun-block in some suncreams, and large doses may be used in the treatment of skin disorders.

parboil A way of tenderizing foods by boiling them for a short time. Some vegetables, such as French beans and mangetout, may be parboiled and then chilled to be used in salads. Others, such as potatoes, may be parboiled to soften them prior to roasting. Parboiling causes some losses of vitamins and minerals through **leaching**, and some reduction of vitamins that are unstable at boiling point (e.g. **pantothenic acid**, **thiamin** and **vitamin C**). Parboiling of beans before using them in salads ensures that harmful **phytic acid** and **lectins** are destroyed. See also **blanching**.

parsley A small herbaceous European plant, the curly, aromatic leaves of which are used as a herb and garnish. Parsley is eaten in small quantities but its nutritional properties should not be ignored. It is high in **dietary fibre**, provides some **protein** and is very rich in **potassium**, **carotene** and **vitamin C**. Although rich in **calcium** and **iron**, the amount available to the body is probably small because of the presence of **oxalic acid**. Parsley is believed to stimulate the appetite, aid digestion and act as a mild diuretic. Dried parsley has a much lower vitamin C content than fresh parsley.

parsnip A long white-fleshed root vegetable. Parsnips provide **starch**, and **dietary fibre** (includ-

ing **pectin**), and some **protein** and **sugars**. They
have an energy value of 56 kcal/100 g (boiled parsnip). Parsnips also contain useful amounts of **folic acid** and small amounts of **iron**, **thiamin**, **niacin**, **pantothenic acid** and **vitamin C**.

partridge A small **game** bird usually cooked by
roasting. Partridge provides **protein** and some **fat**,
and has an energy value of 212 kcal/100 g (roast
meat). It is high in **sodium**, **potassium**, **phosphorus**,
iron and **sulphur**.

passion flower See **passion fruit tea**.

passion fruit A small, wrinkled, olive green or
black tropical fruit with sweet, fragrant white
flesh containing tiny black seeds. Because the
seeds are eaten together with the flesh, passion
fruit has a high **dietary fibre** content. It provides
sugars, small amounts of **protein**, **vitamin C**, **potassium**, **magnesium** and **phosphorus**, and has an
energy value of 34 kcal/100 g.

passion fruit tea (or **passion flower tea**) A delicately perfumed tea made from the fruits and or
flowers of the passion fruit popular for its soothing qualities.

pasta (or **noodles**) A dough traditionally made
from refined white wheat flour or semolina and
water (and sometimes eggs and milk), moulded
into a number of characteristic shapes, e.g. spa-

ghetti, lasagne, tagliatelle, macaroni, and sold fresh or dried. Pasta is high in **starch**, provides some **protein** and has an energy value of 117 kcal/100 g (boiled). Wholemeal pasta has a grainy texture and is brown in colour. It contains more **dietary fibre**, minerals and **B complex vitamins** than white pasta. Dyeing pasta, traditionally with spinach water, does not change the nutritional value. Fresh pasta usually contains eggs and milk, which increase the protein, calcium and thiamin contents. Canned pasta in tomato sauce may be made with refined or wholewheat flour. It has an energy value of 59 kcal/100 g and a higher **sodium** content than fresh or dried pasta.

pasteurization A mild form of heat treatment, named after its inventor, Louis Pasteur (1822–1895), used to destroy bacteria in foods and to increase the keeping quality of foods. Pasteurization is used for foods such as milk, beer and fruit juices. Milk is heated to about 70°C for 15 seconds. This process does not stop milk from souring but it does kill bacteria which might cause disease. Pasteurization of milk causes a 10% loss of the **B complex vitamins** thiamin, pyridoxine, folic acid and vitamin B_{12}, and a 25% loss of **vitamin C**. See also **ultra heat treated**.

pastry A dough made from flour, water and fat (e.g. vegetable oil, butter, suet) which may include other ingredients such as eggs, sugar or cheese. Pastry is high in **starch** and contains varying amounts of **fat**, and therefore varying energy values. Cooked shortcrust pastry has an energy value of 527 kcal/100 g, flaky pastry a value of 565 kcal/100 g and choux pastry a value of 330 kcal/100 g. Depending on the type of fat used, the pastry will contain proportionately more or less **saturated fatty acids**. Pastry made with wholemeal flour provides more **dietary fibre**, minerals and **B complex vitamins** than pastry made with white, refined flour.

paté A savoury paste made from finely ground meat, poultry, offal, fish or vegetable matter. Patés have different nutritional values according to their ingredients. In general, they provide **protein** and a high level of **fat** and have correspondingly high energy values, although low-fat varieties are also available. Patés tend to be salty, which means they have a high **sodium** content, and they often contain **nitrates** and **nitrites** as preservatives.

pawpaw See **papaya**.

pea A general name for the seed of certain **pulses**, including the chickpea and the garden pea. The name is usually applied to the small, characteristically bright green seed of the garden pea, which is eaten cooked as a vegetable. The unripe seed pod is also edible (see **mangetout**). Garden peas provide more **protein**, **sugars**, **starch** and **dietary fibre** than most other common vegetables, and have a correspondingly higher energy value of 52 kcal/100 g (boiled, fresh or frozen). They also contain **calcium**, **iron**, **vitamin C**, **thiamin**, **riboflavin** and **niacin**, and some **molybdenum** and **manganese**. None of these micronutrients are seriously depleted in frozen or canned garden peas, but almost all of the vitamin C and much of the B complex vitamin content is lost in canned processed (mushy) peas. Dried peas and split dried peas, which may be soaked and cooked like fresh peas or soaked to make sprouts, contain only a small percentage of the vitamin C content of fresh peas. Like all pulses, peas may contain some **phytic acid** and toxic **lectins**. They should be thoroughly cooked or sprouted for several days to break down these harmful substances.

peach A red apple-sized fruit with delicate, slightly furry skin and sweet, tender yellow or white flesh. Peaches contain some **sugars**, have an energy value of 37 kcal/100 g and provide reasonable amounts of **carotene**, **niacin** and **potassium**. Dried peaches keep most of their nutritional value. Canned peaches, if sweetened, contain more sugars and have a higher energy value of 87 kcal/100 g. Up to 50% of the carotene and niacin content is lost during the canning process.

peanut (also called **groundnut** or **monkey nut**) The seed (not in fact a nut) of a small leguminous bush that pushes its thin, woody fruit capsules below ground as they mature. Peanuts are a major food crop, processed into cattle feed and oils, as well as the familiar, salted snack. Rich in **protein** and **fat**, of which a high proportion is monounsaturated **fatty acid**, they also provide reasonable amounts of **dietary fibre**, **sugars** and **starch**. They have a high energy value of 570 kcal/100 g. Peanuts also contain **potassium**, **calcium**, **magnesium**, **molybdenum**, **manganese**, **sulphur**, **thiamin**, **niacin**, **vitamin E**, **folic acid** and **pantothenic acid**, and small amounts of **zinc**, **iron** and **vitamin B_6**. Like most pulses, raw peanuts contain some **phytic acid** and toxic **lectins**, but these substances are broken down or destroyed by roasting, cooking or sprouting. Salted peanuts have a very high **sodium** content and roasted peanuts contain less thiamin and no folic acid.

peanut butter A rich, oily paste made from crushed peanuts. It has a high **fat** content, and provides **protein**, **dietary fibre**, **starch** and some **sugars**, as well as most of the vitamins and minerals associated with the **peanut** (but the sulphur content is eliminated and the levels of thiamin, vitamin E, folic acid and pantothenic acid are lower). These nutritional losses are slightly less in the 'crunchy' variety, which contains chopped peanuts, than in the 'smooth' variety. Like peanuts, peanut butter may contain small amounts of **phytic acid** and **lectins**. Peanut butter almost always contains added salt and, therefore, has a high **sodium** content. It may also contain added sugar, preservatives and colouring.

pear A rounded or elongated bell-shaped fruit with thin yellow, green or pinkish skin and juicy, sweet white flesh that has a characteristically grainy texture. The pear contains small amounts of **sugars** and **dietary fibre**, and has an energy value of 41 kcal/100 g. It contains only a little **vitamin C** and makes a negligible contribution to micronutrient intakes.

pearl barley Seeds of barley from which the germ or embryo and the outer bran have been removed. Pearl barley is high in **starch** and has an energy value of 360 kcal/100 g. It contains small amounts of **phosphorus, zinc, niacin, vitamin E, vitamin B₆, folic acid** and **pantothenic acid**, but much of the **B complex vitamin** content is destroyed in cooking.

pecan nut The smooth, dark red nut of the pecan tree. The slightly bitter, oily kernel looks and tastes rather like a walnut. It is high in **fat**, with a high proportion of **unsaturated fatty acids** and has a correspondingly high energy value of 696 kcal/100 g. Pecan nuts provide some **protein** and small amounts of **iron, zinc, manganese** and **B complex vitamins**.

pectin A non-starch **polysaccharide** present in fruit and vegetables, particularly root vegetables such as parsnips, swedes, turnips and yams. Pectin forms a stiff gel under certain conditions and this property is important in jam making, and explains the use of pectin as a gelling agent in a number of manufactured foods. Pectin lowers levels of **cholesterol** in the blood and reduces **blood glucose** (see **diabetes**).

pellagra The disease characteristic of **niacin** deficiency. The symptoms at the onset of the disease include weakness, loss of weight, a sore tongue, mental confusion, depression and a redness of the skin on the exposed parts of the body. Severe cases involve three conditions, dermatitis, diarrhoea and dementia. All these symptoms are due to derangements of the digestive system, skin and brain cells. Pellagra occurs in communities where the diet consists largely of maize. In the UK it only occurs as a result of an underlying disease such as alcoholism.

pepper, black or white A hot-tasting powder made by grinding whole **peppercorns** at different stages of maturity and used for seasoning and adding pungency to foods. Black pepper is made from peppercorns picked before they are quite ripe and dried in the sun, where they blacken in a day or two. White pepper is made from ripened peppercorns that have been soaked and rubbed to remove their husks. Pepper is a good source of **copper**, but it is consumed in such small quantities that its nutritional contents are virtually negligible. See also **chilli pepper**.

peppercorn The dried fruit of the tropical, climbing vine native to India. Peppercorns are used whole or powdered as a spice. See **pepper, black or white**.

peppers (also called **pimientos** or **sweet peppers**) Crisp green (unripe), red, yellow or orange fruits of a species of **capsicum**. Peppers are very good sources of **vitamin C** and **carotene**, although the vitamin C content is depleted in cooking. They have low energy values of 15 kcal/ 100 g.

peppermint tea A refreshing infusion made from the leaves of the peppermint plant. Mint contains menthol, which may have a number of beneficial effects on the digestive system, such as stimulating the appetite.

peptides Intermediate products of **protein** digestion that are further broken down by enzymes to **amino acids**.

persimmon The large, sweet, orange-red fruit of a hard-wooded tropical tree. Persimmons provide **sugars** and small amounts of **dietary fibre** and **protein**. They also contain **vitamin C** and **carotene**.

pesticides Chemical products sprayed over fruit, cereals and vegetables to protect them from insects (insecticides) and fungi (fungicides). Almost 99% of all crops are sprayed with insecticides and this means that many meat and dairy products also contain pesticides because the

plants used as fodder for stock are sprayed. Long-
term consumption of even small quantities of
some pesticides may cause birth defects, cancer
and other degenerative diseases. The Ministry of
Agriculture, Foods and Fisheries and the Department of Health have banned one notorious health
risk, DDT, and have imposed restrictions on the
use of other pesticides to maintain safe levels of
these substances in food. Fruits contain the highest levels of pesticides; these levels may be lowered
by peeling the fruits (although, in fruits such
as apples, which are usually eaten with their peel,
this will cause some loss of dietary fibre and vitamins and minerals) or washing them, especially if
a small amount of vinegar is added to the water.
Vegetables should also be washed. Most forms of
cooking, particularly boiling, will break down the
chemicals used in pesticides (but this will, of
course, also break down some of the vitamin
content). Many people now look for organically
grown fruits, vegetables and cereals. Organic
foods are grown in the absence of artificial
pesticides and fertilizers, and are available at
most health food shops and large supermarkets.

pH A measure of the acidity or alkalinity of a
liquid. PH stands for potential hydrogen and
refers to the proportion of available hydrogen units in a liquid. The scale ranges from 0 (very
acid) to 14 (very alkaline). Distilled water has a
pH value of 7 (neutral).

pheasant A long-tailed **game** bird whose flesh is usually cooked by roasting, or in pies and patés. It is high in **protein** and low in **fat**, and has an energy value of 213 kcal/100 g. It also provides some **potassium**, **calcium**, **magnesium**, **phosphorus** and, like other game, is a particularly good source of well-absorbed **iron**.

phospholipid Fatty substances made up of **glycerol**, **phosphorus** and up to two **fatty acids** that are concerned with the transport of fat in the bloodstream. They are widespread in plant and animal foods, as part of the structure of cells, but dietary supplies are unnecessary as the body makes its own phospholipids.

phosphorus A non-metallic mineral, second only to calcium in abundance in the body (the average adult male body contains about 700 g of phosphorus). Phosphorus is vital to the formation of strong bones and teeth and it plays an important role in the release and storage of energy in the body. It is a key constituent of the sheath that protects the nerve fibres, and it helps maintain the correct **pH** balance in different parts of the body. Good sources of phosphorus are cheese, liver, lentils, wholegrain bread, eggs, meat, fish, milk and yeast extract, but it is found in all foods with the exception of fats, oils and sugar. There is no UK **RDA**. The US RDA is 800 mg a day, but diets that contain sufficient protein and calcium contain enough phosphorus. Deficiency of phosphorus alone from an inadequate diet does not occur in humans. Temporary inadequacies in the diet are counteracted by the kidneys cutting down the amount they excrete. Excess phosphorus is probably harmless for adults. It is either not absorbed or is eliminated by the kidneys.

phytic acid A compound of **inositol** and **phosphorus**, found chiefly in wholegrain cereals, nuts and pulses. It readily combines with essential minerals (e.g. calcium, iron, magnesium and zinc) during digestion and inhibits their absorption by the body. The body can adapt to a high phytic acid intake in the diet by increasing the amount of phytase, an enzyme present in the intestine, so that after a time the binding effect of phytic acid is reduced. Phytic acid is also broken down by enzymes in yeast during proving and baking of bread, and in pulses when they are soaked in water. Unleavened bread such as pitta bread and some pizzas contain phytic acid.

pickles Foods, usually vegetables (such as onions or gherkins), that have been preserved in vinegar or brine, or spicy sauces made from fruit and/or vegetables. Pickles tend to have a high acidity because of their vinegar content, and they usually have a high **sodium** content. Pickled foods have similar nutritional values to their fresh ingredients, but much of the **vitamin C** and **pantothenic acid** contents may be lost during storing.

pickling The preservation of foods such as vegetables and fish in **acetic acid** or **lactic acid**. Pure acetic acid may be used but more commonly it is used, in the form of vinegar.

pigeon A small **game** bird usually cooked by roasting or served in pies. Pigeons provide **protein** and some **fat**, and have an energy value of 230 kcal/100 g (roast meat). They are a remarkably rich source of well-absorbed **iron**, and a good source of **sodium**, **potassium**, **phosphorus**, **sulphur** and **niacin**.

pilchard A small saltwater fish eaten fresh or canned in oil or tomato sauce. Pilchards provide **protein** and are a good source of **calcium**, **iron**, **zinc** and **vitamin B$_{12}$**. They also contain smaller amounts of **potassium**, **magnesium** and **phosphorus**, and have a high **sodium** content. Pilchards canned in tomato sauce have an energy value of 230 kcal/100 g, but the fat content and corresponding energy value is much higher if they are fried or canned in oil.

pimientos See **peppers**.

pineapple A large tropical fruit with tough, scratchy skin and fibrous, juicy, yellow flesh. Pineapples provide **sugars** (unusually mostly as sucrose), are a good source of **vitamin C**, and contain some **potassium** and **magnesium**. Canned pineapples have only half the potassium, magnesium and vitamin C content of the fresh fruit. Fresh pineapple has an energy value of 46 kcal/ 100 g. Pineapple canned in syrup contains nearly twice the sugar content and has an energy value of 77 kcal/100 g. Pineapples contain bromelain, an enzyme that digests protein, which is sometimes used to tenderize meat.

Pineapple juice contains sugars, has an energy value of 53 kcal/100 g and provides potassium, but less vitamin C than fresh pineapple, or grapefruit, orange and tomato juice.

pineapple juice   See **pineapple**.

pine kernel   The oily, aromatic seed of certain varieties of pine tree. Pine kernels are often roasted and sprinkled over desserts or salads to add flavour and texture. They have a high **fat** content, with a high proportion of monounsaturated **fatty acids**, and also provide some **dietary fibre** and small amounts of **starch**, **sugars** and **protein**. Pine kernels have an energy value of 642 kcal/100 g. They provide some **B complex vitamins** and **vitamin E**.

pistachio nut   The characteristically green, almond-flavoured fruit kernel of a small western Asian tree. It is related to the cashew nut. Pistachio nuts may be eaten fresh or roasted or used to flavour foods such as ice cream. They are rich in **fat**, with a high proportion of monounsaturated **fatty acids** and a correspondingly high energy value of 626 kcal/100 g. They provide **protein** and some **dietary fibre**, **iron**, **calcium**, **phosphorus**, **potassium**, **manganese** and small amounts of most **B complex vitamins** and some **vitamin E**. Pistachio nuts are usually sold salted and, therefore, have a high **sodium** content.

pitta bread A flat, rounded, only slightly leavened bread. Pitta bread may be made with refined white or wholewheat flour. The whole-wheat variety provides more **dietary fibre**. Because pitta bread is only partly leavened it may contain some ´phytic acid´. It has an energy value of 257 kcal/100 g for white and 236 kcal/100 g for wholemeal pitta bread.

pizza A disc of dough usually topped with tomatoes, cheese and a variety of other ingredients. The dough base may be made from wholewheat or refined flour and it may be thick and bread-like or unleavened (see **phytic acid**). The nutritional content and energy value of a pizza depends on the amount of oil and on the ingredients used in its topping.

plaice A white flat fish. Plaice provides protein, a low **fat** content and a correspondingly low energy value of 93 kcal/100 g (steamed). It also contains good sources of **potassium**, **thiamin**, **vitamin B_6** and **pantothenic acid**. Baking, steaming, grilling and frying cause little loss of nutrients.

plantain A variety of large banana, that is cooked and eaten when green (sometimes called the 'cooking banana'). Plantains have a high **starch** content, provide some **dietary fibre**, small amounts of **protein** and have an energy value of 122 kcal/100 g (boiled). They contain negligible amounts of **micronutrients**. Plantains may be steamed or roasted.

plum A small fruit, of which there are many varieties, with a thin skin (that may be purple, green or yellow, with or without red patches) and sweet fibrous yellow or pinkish flesh. Plums provide **sugars**, dessert plums have a higher sugar content than plums grown for cooking or canning, and a small amount of **protein** and **dietary fibre**. Fresh plums have an energy value of 38 kcal/100 g, those stewed with sugar a value of 59 kcal/100 g. They contain **potassium** and **carotene** but very little **vitamin C**. See also **prunes**.

PMT See **premenstrual syndrome**.

polysaccharides Complex **carbohydrates** that either function as storage polysaccharides, such as **starch** and **glycogen**, or as structural polysaccharides in plant cell walls, such as **cellulose**, **pectin** and **gums**. From a dietary point of view, storage polysaccharides are used for energy supply and structural polysaccharides contribute to **dietary fibre** intake.

polyunsaturated fatty acid (also called **PUFA** or **polyunsaturate**) A fatty acid with four or more hydrogen atoms missing and therefore two or more double bonds. Polyunsaturated fatty acids have been found to lower the blood **cholesterol** level. However, they are less effective in lowering the cholesterol level than **saturated fatty acids** are in raising it. They reduce the blood cholesterol by speeding up the process by which it is eliminated by the **bile**. Polyunsaturated fatty acids are found mainly in vegetable oils, cereal grains and fish, although not all vegetable oils are good sources. Lean meat can also provide useful amounts of polyunsaturated fatty acids. To ensure a lower level of cholesterol in the blood, it is better to reduce the total **fat** content of the diet than to raise the proportion of polyunsaturated to saturated fats.

pomegranate A round tropical fruit with hard reddish skin and juicy pink flesh made up of many small, crisp seed-bearing pods. The pomegranate contains **sugars**, and provides reasonable amounts of **potassium**, but little **vitamin C**. It has an energy value of 44 kcal/100 g. Grenadine syrup, a cordial popular in France, is made from pomegranate juice.

poppy seed The tiny black seed of the poppy used to decorate bread and desserts. Poppy seeds are rich in **polyunsaturated fatty acids** and contain reasonable amounts of other nutrients, but they are used in such small quantities that their nutritional values are negligible.

pork Pig meat. Pork tends to have a fairly high **fat** content, with a high proportion of **saturated fatty acids**, but the fat content can be reduced by stripping away visible fat from the lean meat. For instance grilled belly of pork has an energy value of 398 kcal/100 g and that of lean roast pork 185 kcal/100 g. Pork provides **protein** and is a good source of **zinc**, **thiamin**, **riboflavin**, **niacin**, and **vitamin B₆**. It also contains smaller amounts of **potassium**, **magnesium**, **phosphorus**, **iron**, and **selenium**. See also **bacon**; **ham**.

porridge A smooth paste made with oat flakes soaked and cooked in water and/or milk, and usually eaten hot at breakfast time. Porridge provides the nutrients associated with **oats** (**starch**, **protein**, **B complex vitamins** and **minerals**). The use of milk, whole, semi-skimmed or skimmed, and sugar will affect the energy value and nutritional composition of the porridge.

port A deep red, sweet, fortified dessert wine originally from Portugal, and available in different colours, strengths and vintages. Port contains between 18 and 20% **alcohol** by volume. It has a fairly high sugar content and has an energy value of 157 kcal/100 g.

potassium A mineral found in the fluids within cells and essential for healthy cell function. In conjunction with **sodium**, it regulates the levels of acidity and alkalinity in the body, and helps maintain the correct water balance. It is an important factor in the functioning of nerves and muscles. Potassium is found in nearly all foods except sugar, fats and oils, but particularly good sources include green leafy vegetables, mushrooms, bananas, potatoes, grapes, tomatoes and brewer's yeast. There are no losses on baking and steaming but boiling vegetables can cause up to 50% loss, although this can be recovered in the cooking water. Potassium deficiency due to inadequate intake is rare in healthy adults and children. Nearly all the 2–6 g of potassium in the average daily diet is absorbed into the bloodstream and adequately replaces body losses. Deficiency can be caused by prolonged diarrhoea or repeated vomiting (these may be induced in **bulimia nervosa**) or by regular use of **diuretics** (particularly in the elderly). Symptoms of potassium deficiency are weakness, mental confusion and, in severe cases, heart attack. There is no harmful level of potassium intake in a healthy adult, because any excess is removed by the kidneys.

potato A starchy, white tuber eaten as a vegetable. Potatoes consist mainly of water and **starch** with a little **protein** and **dietary fibre**. Potatoes are an important source of **vitamin C** (especially in winter) and they supply 20% of the total intake in the average UK diet. The vitamin C content is highest in new potatoes and it decreases if the potatoes are stored, and some of it is lost in cooking. They also contain **potassium**, **thiamin**, **niacin**

and **vitamin B₆**. The energy value of potatoes varies depending on the way they are cooked. Chips and roast potatoes have higher energy values (253 kcal/100 g and 157 kcal/100 g respectively) than boiled or baked potatoes (80 kcal/100 g and 105 kcal/100 g respectively). If potatoes are not stored correctly in a dark, dry, cool place they develop green patches which contain a toxic substance, solanine. Solanine also appears when old potatoes begin to sprout. It should be avoided, as it causes nausea, vomiting and abdominal pain.

poultry The meat of domestic fowl such as **chicken**, **duck** and **turkey**. Poultry flesh is relatively low in **fat** when compared with red meats with most of the fat content in the skin. The nutritional content and energy value of poultry varies, but they all provide **protein**.

prawn Characteristically pink, mild-tasting shellfish. Prawns contain **protein**, no **carbohydrate** and very little **fat**. They have an energy value of 107 kcal/100 g (boiled), a very high **sodium** content and provide **calcium**, **phosphorus**, **copper**, **iodine**, **sulphur** and **niacin**.

premenstrual syndrome (also called **premenstrual tension** or **PMT**) A variety of unpleasant and often uncomfortable symptoms experienced by many women in the days immediately preceding menstruation. Symptoms vary according to the individual, but they tend to include irritability, tiredness and depression, headaches, back ache, cramps in the lower abdomen, tenderness of the breasts, acne and water retention (see **oedema**). These symptoms may be alleviated by ensuring a high dietary intake of **calcium**, **magnesium**, **selenium**, **vitamin B₆** and **vitamin E**, or by taking supplements of these micronutrients. **Evening primrose oil** has been found to reduce or eliminate some or all of the symptoms in many individuals.

premenstrual tension See **premenstrual syndrome**.

preservatives A variety of substances used as food additives to prevent spoilage, particularly by inhibiting bacterial growth. Manufacturers may only add the preservatives permitted by law. The laws governing food-labelling oblige manufacturers to name preservatives among the ingredients. Commonly used preservatives include sulphur dioxides and benzoates, which are mostly used on fruits, vegetables and fruit and vegetable products; **nitrites**, which are used mostly in meat products; and propionic acid, which is used in bread, cakes and pastries. Some natural substances may be used as preservatives, e.g. vinegar in pickles, sugar in preserves and salt in salted meat and fish.

pressure cooking A method of **boiling** under pressure, in which higher temperatures are used but cooking time is reduced. The nutritive value remains much the same as in boiling, and it may occasionally be better as more **vitamin C** and **B complex vitamins** are retained.

protein Essential components of all living matter, made up of long chains of individual units called **amino acids**. The cells of our bones, muscles, skin, nails, hair and every other tissue are made up of proteins, as are vital fluids such as blood, enzymes and hormones. Protein is constantly being broken down and replaced. In food it is broken down into its component amino acids during digestion, then absorbed and rearranged into new body protein. Of the 20 or so amino acids, 8 are called essential amino acids because they cannot be synthesized by the body and must be obtained from foods. Foods that contain all eight of these substances in the proportions required by the body are said to provide high-quality proteins. High-quality proteins are usually found in animal foods such as eggs, milk and other dairy products, fish and meat. Some plant sources contain high-quality proteins: tofu, soya beans (sprouted or not), corn, peas, peanuts, wheat germ and brewer's yeast. **Vegans** often combine different plant food proteins at a meal so that the amino acids complement each other.

RDA for protein represents 10% of the energy requirement. This level ensures a palatable diet and adequate provision of other nutrients that tend to accompany protein in foods, but people can consume much smaller quantities and still retain health. There is little evidence to suggest that eating too much protein is a health risk, although a diet consistently high in animal protein has been linked to constipation and even cancer of the colon. A diet low in protein is particularly harmful in the young who are still growing. In adults, a protein deficiency causes poor skin, nail and hair condition, even hair loss as non-essential protein replacement ceases. Later, muscles waste as amino acids from the muscle proteins are used to make more vital proteins such as enzymes. The liver accumulates fat and blood proteins are not replaced.

provitamin   A substance that the body can use to synthesize vitamins, or which it converts into vitamins. The most common pro-vitamins are **carotene**, which can be converted into **vitamin A**, and a derivative of **cholesterol** in the skin, which is converted into **vitamin D** by the action of ultraviolet rays.

prune   A dried plum. Traditionally prunes are dried on the tree, but nowadays they are more likely to be artificially dried. Prunes provide **sugars**, a good source of **dietary fibre** and have an energy value of 82 kcal/100 g (stewed without sugar). They also contain **potassium** and are a reasonable source of **carotene**. Prunes have a mild laxative effect because of the high concentration of dietary fibre and the presence of a substance called diphenylisatin.

PUFA See **polyunsaturated fatty acid**.

pulses (also called **legumes**) The edible seeds of leguminous plants such as beans, peas and lentils. Pulses are good sources of **protein**, and also provide **sugars, starch** and **dietary fibre**. With the exception of soya, they are low in **fat**. They are rich in **calcium, thiamin, riboflavin** and **niacin**, and also contain some **iron, molybdenum, manganese** and **carotene**. If they are washed and soaked for a few days, many pulses can be eaten as sprouts, which have the additional benefit of being rich in **vitamin C**. See individual entries for energy values. The seed pods of some leguminous plants (**French beans, mangetout** and **runner beans**) are eaten when they are unripe and the seeds are only very small. They, therefore, provide proportionally less of the above nutrients and more dietary fibre. Most pulses contain small amounts of **phytic acid** and toxic **lectins**, which are broken down when the pulses are cooked or sprouted. See also **adzuki bean; beans; broad bean; butter bean; chickpea; dahls; haricot bean; kidney bean; lentil; mung bean; peanut; pea; soya bean**.

pumpernickel A dark, grainy nutritious bread made entirely with **rye**.

pumpkin The large round fruit of a plant of American origin related to the cucumber, with a tough orange rind and pulpy orange flesh. The flesh of the pumpkin has a very high water content with a correspondingly low energy value of 15 kcal/100 g and only small amounts of **protein, carbohydrate** and **dietary fibre**. It is a good source of **carotene**.

pumpkin seed The smooth, green nutritious seed of the pumpkin. Pumpkin seeds are sprinkled over food to add flavour and texture. They are rich in **fat**, with a high proportion of **polyunsaturated fatty acids**, and a high energy value of 610 kcal/100 g. Pumpkin seeds are also rich in **protein**.

pyridoxine See **vitamin B₆**.

quail A small **game** bird. Quail provides **protein**, is low in **fat** and has an energy value of 132 kcal/100 g (raw flesh, no skin). It also contains some **phosphorus, calcium** and **magnesium**, and small amounts of **B complex vitamins**. It is usually cooked by roasting.

quiche A savoury tart with a pastry case and a filling of eggs, milk and a selection of other ingredients, which may include meat, poultry, fish and vegetables. The nutritional content and energy value of a quiche varies according to its ingredients. Regardless of the other ingredients, the combination of eggs and milk means that quiches contain **protein, potassium, calcium, iron, zinc, vitamin A, B complex vitamins, vitamin D** and **vitamin E**.

quince A pear-shaped hard fruit with thin yellow skin and white flesh that is too acidic to eat raw. Quinces are used in preserves and fruity sauces. They contain large quantities of **pectin**, as well as **sugars**, **dietary fibre**, **potassium** and small amounts of **vitamin C**. They have an energy value of 25 kcal/100 g.

rabbit A small, long-eared, herbivorous **game** mammal usually served in casseroles and stews. The nutritional content of its white meat is similar to the dark meat of a chicken. It contains **protein**, only a small amount of **fat** and has an energy value of 179 kcal/100 g (stewed). It is a good source of **niacin** and **vitamin** B_{12} and provides smaller amounts of **iron**, **zinc**, **phosphorus**, **riboflavin**, **thiamin** and **vitamin** B_6.

radish A small rounded root with pink skin and pungent white flesh, eaten in salads. Radishes have a very high water content, very little **protein** and **sugars** and no **fat**, and an energy value of 15 kcal/100 g. They also contain small amounts of **iron**, **copper**, **vitamin C** and **folic acid**. The long white mooli is also a type of radish with a similar nutritional composition.

raising agent A mixture of an acid and alkali that produces carbon dioxide gas in cakes, biscuits, scones and soda bread. The usual alkali is bicarbonate of soda and the acid, tartaric acid. When mixed with water or put into a hot oven, carbon dioxide is released and expands causing the mixture to rise. Because bicarbonate of soda breaks down **vitamin B₁**, in proportion to the amount used, **yeast** should be used to raise bread.

raisin A dried black grape. Raisins are rich in **sugars**, good sources of **dietary fibre** and have an energy value of 246 kcal/100 g. They provide **potassium, magnesium, iron, copper, zinc, sulphur, thiamin** and **vitamin B₆**. Because **mineral hydrocarbons** are often added to raisins they should be washed before eating.

rape-seed oil A vegetable oil extracted from the seeds of the yellow-flowered rape plant and used for cooking and dressings. Rape-seed oil contains a high proportion of unsaturated **fatty acids** and has an energy value of 899 kcal/100 g.

raspberry A small, red fruit of the raspberry shrub made up of many tiny, soft pods round a white core. The raspberry has a very high water content and provides less sugar than most other fruits. It has an energy value of 25 kcal/100 g. Raspberries contain significant amounts of **vitamin C** and smaller amounts of **iron, copper, potassium, pantothenic acid** and **biotin**. Frozen raspberries are as good nutritionally as the fresh fruit, but some of the copper, most of the vitamin C and pantothenic acid and all of the biotin is lost in canned raspberries. Canned, sweetened raspberries have a higher energy value of 87 kcal/100 g.

raspberry leaf tea An infusion made from the leaves of the raspberry plant. It contains fragarine, which suppresses contractions of the uterus. Raspberry leaf tea is often recommended to soothe the cramps some women experience in premenstrual syndrome.

RDA (also called **recommended daily amount**, **recommended daily allowance**, **recommended daily intake** or **RDI**) The average quantity or amount of food energy, protein, vitamins and minerals that should be provided per head in a group of people if the needs of practically all members of the group are to be met. Actual requirements vary considerably according to age, sex and occupation; they are also affected by illness, pregnancy, lactation, stress and physical exertion.

The RDA of any nutrient varies from country to country depending on the criteria by which it has been established, and it should only be used as a guideline. If a diet is deficient in vitamins and minerals, foods rich in the deficient micronutrients should be included in the diet. Vitamins and minerals can also be obtained from supplements and from fortified or enriched foods. The RDAs of vitamins and minerals quoted in this book are the UK RDA, established by the Department of Health. Where there is no UK RDA, the US RDA has been quoted. For individual requirements see entries for the different nutrients and micronutrients.

RDI See **RDA**.

recommended daily allowance See **RDA**.

recommended daily intake See **RDA**.

redcurrant A small, round, shiny red fruit, which grows in bunches and is related to the gooseberry and blackcurrant. Redcurrants are a good source of **dietary fibre**, provide small amounts of **sugars** and **protein**, and have an energy value of 21 kcal/100 g. They also contain some **vitamin C**, although only 20% of that found in blackcurrants. Redcurrants contain smaller amounts of **potassium**, **iron**, **carotene** and **biotin**, but some of the biotin and about half of the vitamin C are lost if redcurrants are stewed. The seedlings of the redcurrant, known as white currants, have a slightly different flavour and no carotene content.

reduced-calorie (products) Foods that have had their energy value reduced. This is usually achieved by adding water, extracting some of the **fat** (for example, skimming milk), by cooking processed foods in less fat or reducing the sugar content. Artificial **sweeteners** with no energy value may be added to replace sugar.

relish One of a number of spicy sauces, usually made from fruits or vegetables. The nutritional and energy values vary according to the ingredients, but most of them have a high **sodium** content, from salt addition, are slightly acidic because

204

of the addition of vinegar and contain sugar. These ingredients are added for flavour and for their preserving actions

retinol   The chemical name for **vitamin A**. Vitamin A can also be obtained from **carotene**. In general, retinol is found in animal foods and carotene is found in plant foods.

rhubarb   The crisp, pink, sour stalk of the rhubarb plant. It has a very high water content, contains only small amounts of **sugars**, **dietary fibre** and **protein**, and has an energy value of 6 kcal/100 g (stewed). It also contains only small amounts of **vitamin C** and negligible amounts of other **micronutrients**. It contains relatively large amounts of **calcium** but this is combined with **oxalic acid** and so is not easily absorbed by the body. Rhubarb leaves should not be eaten because they contain toxic levels of oxalic acid. Rhubarb is very bitter and is usually stewed and sweetened, this raises the energy value to 45 kcal/100 g.

riboflavin (also known as **vitamin B$_2$**)   One of the **B complex vitamins** needed for growth and for the maintenance of healthy skin and eyes. It is essential for the release of energy from food. It is found in nearly all foods, but particularly good sources are yeast extract, brewer's yeast, liver, soya beans, dairy products, wheat bran and eggs. Riboflavin is fairly stable to heat, but is destroyed by ultraviolet light. Losses during cooking are usually caused by **leaching** and these can be reduced by using the cooking water for gravies or sauces. The required amount of riboflavin is affected by the number of active cells (all but fat cells) and because in general men have more muscle and less fat than women the **RDA** is 1.6 mg for men and 1.3 mg for women. Although a deficiency does not appear to have any serious effects, it may contribute to cracking of the lips and corners of the mouth, inflammation of the tongue, sore and itchy eyes and dry or scaly skin on parts of the face. However, none of these symtoms are specific to riboflavin deficiency.

rice A cereal that is the staple food in many Asian countries. Rice has a lower **protein** content than other cereals, is a good source of most **B complex vitamins** and has an energy value of 123 kcal/100 g. It is chiefly eaten as polished or white rice, which has most of the B complex vitamins removed. In brown rice only the outer husk is removed and it retains most of the **micronutrients** and **dietary fibre** of the wholegrain.

rickets A disorder that affects babies and children, causing misshapen or soft bones, and characterized by bandy legs and other skeletal changes. Rickets is primarily caused by **vitamin D** deficiency. An important source of vitamin D is the interaction of ultraviolet rays with a derivative of **cholesterol** in the skin, but this process is greatly reduced in certain pigmented skins. Asian children and children who rarely go out into the sun are more likely to develop rickets, and care should be taken to ensure that they consume adequate vitamin D either in foods or as supplements. **Osteomalacia** is the adult form of rickets.

roasting A method of cooking in the oven with radiant heat, or on a spit over or under an open flame. Only those vitamins that are very heat-sensitive, e.g. **vitamin C**, **thiamin** and **pantothenic acid**, are likely to be lost in roasting. Other vitamins may be **leached** into the juices produced during cooking. These juices should be served with the food to minimize such losses. Fat may be added during roasting, which increases the energy value of the roasted food. If the fat is allowed to drip off the food, e.g. when roasting meat on a wire rack, the energy value is reduced.

roe The milt or testis of the male fish (soft roe) and the eggs of the female fish (hard roe). Hard roes contain a high proportion of **protein**, a small amount of **fat**, and have an energy value of 113 kcal/100 g. Soft roes contain less protein and more fat than soft roes and have an energy value of 80 kcal/100 g. Roe, hard and soft, is a rich source of **vitamin A** and **E**, **biotin**, **thiamin** and **copper**. It also contains **vitamins D** and **C** and has a high **cholesterol** level.

rollmop A **herring** fillet pickled in vinegar. Rollmops have a similar nutritional composition to herrings, but have a higher **sodium** content.

rosehip The bright orange-red, berry-like fruit of certain varieties of rose plant. Rosehips, which are rich in **vitamin C** and contain small amounts of **B complex vitamins**. They are used to make syrups and infusions and are traditionally given as nerve tonics and mild laxatives.

rosemary The aromatic grey-green leaves of a small European shrub. Rosemary leaves are used fresh or dried, whole or powdered as a herb. Sprigs of rosemary are used as garnish. It is consumed in such small quantities that its nutritional properties are negligible.

roughage A former term for **dietary fibre**.

royal jelly The milky liquid prepared by worker bees and fed only to the queen bee, causing her to grow to twice the size of a worker, to live up to 50 times as long and to lay up to 2000 eggs a day. Royal jelly is taken as a natural supplement, and is available in pure liquid form, blended with honey or in capsules. It contains high-quality **protein**, **pantothenic acid**, **thiamin**, **riboflavin**, **niacin**, **vitamin B$_6$**, **biotin**, **folic acid**, **vitamin B$_{12}$**, **vitamin C** and **inositol**, as well as **potassium**, **sodium**, **iron**, **chromium**, **manganese** and **nickel**; rich sources for the queen bee but insignificant in the human diet. Royal jelly also contains small amounts of some hormones and enzymes. Many beneficial properties are attributed to it. However, the effects associated with the nutrients and micronutrients it comprises are often exaggerated.

rum A spirit made from molasses. Rum is usually clear (white or silver rum), but it may achieve a rusty brown colour if it is matured in wooden casks (amber rum) or coloured with caramel (demerara rum). The **alcohol** content of rum is usually 37.5% by volume and it has an energy value of 222 kcal/100 ml.

runner bean (also called **string bean**) The fibrous, immature pods of the scarlet runner bean plant; it is a **pulse**. Runner beans have a high water content, contain only small amounts of **protein** and **sugars**, provide some **dietary fibre**, and have an energy value of 19 kcal/100 g (boiled). They are a good source of **carotene**, but the content of most micronutrients is negligible. Runner beans contain **phytic acid** and **lectins** and should not be eaten raw.

rye A cereal that grows in cold climates (an important crop in Scandinavia, the USSR and north Germany). The grain is used to make flour and whisky. Rye flour is high in **starch**, contains small amounts of **protein**, no **dietary fibre** and has an energy value of 321 kcal/100 g. It provides small amounts of **potassium**, **calcium**, **magnesium**, **phosphorus**, **iron**, **copper**, **phosphorus**, molyb-

denum, manganese and **zinc** as well as **thiamin, riboflavin, folic acid** and **biotin**. Rye bread (or pumpernickel) is dark, moist and grainy. It is valued for its vitamin and mineral content, but shoppers should check labels for the percentage of rye in the bread, because many so called rye breads contain mostly refined white flour and only small amounts of rye flour. Crispbreads made using rye flour are popular, nutritious slimming aids in a calorie-controlled diet.

saccharin A **sweetener** that is 300 times sweeter than **sucrose**, and has virtually no energy value. Saccharin, which is characterized by a bitter after-taste, is used commercially and domestically and is available in powder or tablet form.

safflower-seed oil A **vegetable oil** extracted from the safflower-seed and used for cooking and dressings. A deep golden colour in its unrefined state, it is a colourless, flavourless oil when refined. Safflower-seed oil is high in **polyunsaturated fatty acids,** and a rich source of **linoleic acid** (about 75% of its fat content). It has an energy value of 899 kcal/100 g.

saffron The dried yellow-orange stigmas of crocus flowers, used to flavour and colour food. Saffron is consumed in such small quantities that its nutritional properties are negligible.

sage The grey-green leaves of a perennial Mediterranean plant used fresh or dried, whole or powdered, as a herb. Sage is consumed in such small quantities that its nutritional properties are negligible.

sago A cereal obtained from the pithy part of the trunk of the sago palm. It is almost pure **starch** and has an energy value of 355 kcal/100 g, but little other **nutrients** or **micronutrients**. The nutritional deficiencies of sago are overcome when it is cooked with milk.

saithe (also called **coalfish** or **coley**) A white fish. It provides **protein** and small amounts of **potassium**, **sulphur**, **chloride**, **riboflavin**, **niacin**, **vitamin B$_6$** and **vitamin B$_{12}$**. Some of the chloride is lost when saithe is steamed. It has an energy value of 99 kcal/100 g (steamed).

salad dressing An emulsion of oil and vinegar used to coat salad ingredients, such as lettuce leaves, and to give flavour. Most salad dressings (e.g. vinaigrette, salad cream and Thousand Island dressing) have a high energy value, because they contain large proportions of **vegetable oil**. Oil-free and reduced-calorie salad dressings are also available. The nutritional values differ according to their ingredients, for example mayonnaise provides **protein**, **vitamins** and **minerals** because it is made with egg yolks, others may have high **sugar** and **sodium** contents.

salicylate A compound similar to aspirin that occurs naturally in the following foods: most fruits (including dried fruits), some vegetables (chicory, endive, mushrooms, green olives, green peppers, radishes and courgettes), herbs and spices, teas and some coffees, honey, wine and beer. People who have an allergy to aspirin are often also allergic to salicylates. **Hyperactivity** in children is sometimes treated with a salicylate-free diet.

salmon A soft-finned fatty fish native to the Atlantic and Pacific Oceans. Salmon has characteristically pink flesh. It provides **protein**, moderate amounts of **fat** and has an energy value of 197 kcal/100 g (steamed, fresh). Pacific salmon contains **vitamin A**, **vitamin D**, **potassium**, **copper**, **zinc**, **thiamin** and **niacin**, but Atlantic salmon contains no vitamin A and D. Most of the copper and zinc are lost when salmon is cooked or smoked, and smoked salmon is very high in **sodium** and **chloride**; most of the copper and thiamin are lost if it is canned.

salmonella A bacteria that causes food poisoning. Its symptoms are characterized by diarrhoea, vomiting, pains in the abdomen and feverishness. Raw milk, eggs, meat and poultry can be contaminated on the farm or by droppings from pets or pests. It breeds in food at room temperature, but cannot reproduce under refrigeration. It is destroyed by temperatures above 60°C (boiling foods is an effective way of ensuring that it is killed). The incubation period is anything from six hours to two days, depending on the strain and the number of bacteria present. It can take up to a week to recover. Salmonella poisoning should always be diagnosed and treated by a doctor.

salsify A root vegetable valued for its oyster-like flavour. Salsify has a high water content, provides only small amounts of **protein**, minerals and vitamins, and has an energy value of 18 kcal/100 g. It contains no **starch** or **sugars**, but contains inulin (a **polysaccharide** of **fructose**) that has similar properties to **dietary fibre**.

salt (also called **common salt** or **table salt**) A white powder or crystalline solid consisting of sodium chloride and used for seasoning and preserving food. It is the main source of **sodium** in the diet. Salt occurs naturally in foods but it is also added in cooking, at the table and by food manufacturers. Foods that have high salt contents include, canned, smoked, cured or pickled meats; smoked or canned fish, cheese, canned vegetables, breakfast cereals, sauces and soups, yeast extracts, stock cubes, crisps and other savoury snacks. Salt is available as powder or in flakes (sea salt) or crystals (rock salt); there is no significant difference between these different forms. A high consumption of salt is associated with a greater risk of developing **hypertension**, **stroke** and stomach cancer. See also the introductory chapter, A BALANCED DIET.

sardine Small, immature fatty fish of the herring family (usually pilchards), eaten fresh or canned in oil or tomato sauce. Sardines contain **protein** and some **fat**. Sardines canned in oil have an energy value of 217 kcal/100 g and canned in tomato sauce have a value of 177 kcal/100 g. They contain well-absorbed **iron**, **zinc** and **calcium** (from the bones) and are good sources of **vitamin D** and **B$_{12}$**. Sardines have a high **sodium** content. They also provide smaller amounts of **potassium**, **magnesium**, **phosphorus**, **copper**, **sulphur**, **riboflavin**, **niacin**, **vitamin B$_6$**, **pantothenic acid** and **biotin**.

satsuma A small citrus fruit with characteristically loose, bright orange rind and sweet, juicy, orange flesh in crescent-shaped segments, virtually free of pips. Satsumas are related to mandarins and tangerines. They have a high water content, contain very small amounts of **protein**, **sugars** and **dietary fibre**, and have an energy value of 34 kcal/100 g. They also provide some **carotene**, **vitamin C** and **folic acid**.

saturated fatty acids Fatty acids that contain their full quota of hydrogen atoms and have no double bonds. Animal fats and fats that have been hardened, as in the manufacture of most margarine, usually contain more saturated fatty acids than plant and fish oils. The higher the proportion of saturated fatty acids, the more solid the food at room temperature. Foods rich in saturated fatty acids are butter, cream, meat, full-fat milk and eggs. Saturated fatty acids have been found to raise the level of **cholesterol** in the blood and this is associated with **coronary heart disease**. To minimize the risk, it is advisable to reduce the total fat content of the diet and particularly those foods containing a high proportion of saturated fatty acids. See also the introductory chapter, A BALANCED DIET.

sausage   Finely minced or ground meat, often with added fat, mixed with a proportion of crumb, rusk or starch of some kind, seasoned and cased in a skin, traditionally gut but now made from collagen (a protein). The meat is usually pork or beef, often with added offal, gristle and connective tissue. Sausages must contain a certain amount of meat by law, otherwise they cannot be labelled as sausages. Pork sausages must contain 32% lean pork and beef sausages 25% lean beef.

The nutritional value of sausages varies according to the ingredients and the method of cooking, but all sausages are high in fat, with a high proportion of **saturated fatty acids**. Continental sausages, such as salami, have a particularly high fat content. The fat content is increased when sausages are fried rather than grilled. Sausages provide **protein**, some of the **micronutrients** usually associated with meat and high energy values of 318 kcal/100 g (grilled pork) and 491 kcal/100 g (salami). Low-fat varieties, with lower energy values, are also available. All sausages have very high **sodium** contents, and often contain colouring, preservatives, and flavour enhancers such as **monosodium glutamate**.

scurvy   The disease characteristic of **vitamin C** deficiency. Tiredness and depression are the initial symptoms. Over a prolonged period it can cause haemorrhaging, bruising, swollen, bleeding gums, loss of teeth and poor wound healing. Death follows rapidly from internal haemorrhage unless vitamin C is given, when there is a dramatic improvement. Those most at risk are the elderly, the very young and people whose diet contains little or no fresh fruit or vegetables.

seafood stick (also called **crab stick** or **fish stick**)   A characteristically pink and white stick made of fish and used in salads and cooked dishes. They usually contain cod or other white fish and only small amounts, if any, of shellfish. They provide **protein** and very little **fat**. Seafood sticks contain colouring and may also contain preservatives and flavouring.

seakale   Edible shoots of a broad-leaved, European coastal plant. Seakale has a very high water content and an energy value of 7 kcal/100 g, but otherwise its nutritional value is negligible.

seaweed   Marine plants or algae that are cultivated and eaten as vegetables or powdered and sprinkled on food. Seaweeds are one of the few reliable sources of **iodine**, and they have a high **sodium** content. See also **agar**; **alginate**; **kelp**.

seeds The mature, fertilized 'egg' of a plant that usually contains the fertile germ, surrounded by a store of nutrients and a tough outer skin. The nutritional properties of seeds vary according to the species, but in general they provide **protein**, **polyunsaturated fatty acids**, some **dietary fibre**, **sugars** and **starch**, as well as some minerals and vitamins. See **alfalfa**; **poppy seed**; **pulses**; **pumpkin seed**; **sesame seed**; **sunflower seed**.

selenium A **trace element** involved in the body's self-defence mechanisms. Together with **vitamin E** it is part of the **antioxidant** system responsible for preserving the structure and function of cell membranes. Over half the selenium content of the UK diet comes from cereals, especially bread. Other good sources are fish, liver, pork, cheese, eggs, walnuts and brazil nuts. The selenium content of plants depends on the amount of selenium in the soil where they are grown. The requirements for selenium are uncertain but deficiencies have only been reported in areas with poor selenium levels in the soil, such as parts of China and New Zealand. Like other trace elements, selenium is toxic in excess and the safety of supplements is uncertain.

semolina A grainy powder derived from the inner endosperm of grains of hard or durum wheat, a variety of wheat that is high in **gluten**.

Semolina is used to make pasta and is sold as powder to make milk puddings. It is rich in **starch**, provides some **protein** and has an energy value of 350 kcal/100 g. It does not contain significant amounts of any **micronutrients**, but such nutritional deficiencies are overcome when it is cooked with milk.

sesame seed The tiny, oily golden seed of a tropical herbaceous plant of East Indian origin. Sesame seeds are used primarily for flavouring bread and cakes in temperate climates, to make **tahini** or as an ingredient of halva (a Mediterranean sweetmeat). They are rich in **fat**, with a high proportion of **polyunsaturated fatty acids**, and the oil is extracted to make sesame seed oil. The seeds also contain **protein** and have an energy value of 588 kcal/100 g. They contain **iron**, **calcium** and **magnesium**, but little is absorbed because of the presence of **phytic acid**.

sesame seed oil The vegetable oil extracted from the **sesame seed**. It is high in **polyunsaturated fatty acids** (including **linoleic acid**), and an energy value of 899 kcal/100 g. Sesame seed oil also contains some **vitamin E**.

shallot A small bulb related to the onion, with a sweet, intense taste but without being unduly pungent. Shallots are used in cooking to add flavour but should not be browned as this causes them to become bitter. Shallots are high in water with a correspondingly low energy value. They provide only small amounts of **protein** and **sugars**, and negligible amounts of **micronutrients**.

shellfish A general term for edible crustaceans and molluscs. Crustaceans are creatures that have an outer shell (called a carapace) covering the body. Only the flesh of crustaceans is eaten; they include crab, lobster, prawns and shrimps. Molluscs are soft-bodied and usually live inside a hard shell. They tend to be eaten whole, and include cockles, mussels, oysters and winkles (see the individual entries for specific nutritional contents). In general, shellfish are a good source of **protein** and contain virtually no **fat**. Molluscs are sometimes harvested near sewage outflows and may cause food poisoning. It is best, therefore, to buy molluscs from a reliable source. Shellfish should always be bought fresh and cooked (except oysters, which are often eaten raw).

sherry An amber-coloured fortified wine from Spain. Sherry is available in three forms: dry, medium or sweet. These different varieties contain between 13.5 and 17.5% **alcohol** by volume. Their energy value is directly related to the amount of sugar they contain. Sweet sherries have a high sugar content, but some very dry sherries are almost sugar-free and have an energy value of 116 kcal/100 g.

shrimp A general name for many varieties of edible tiny, pink, mild-tasting crustacean shellfish.

Shrimps contain **protein**, very little **fat** and have an energy value of 117 kcal/100 g. They are a good source of **calcium**, **iron**, **iodine** and **zinc**, and also provide smaller amounts of **potassium**, **phosphorus**, **chloride** and **niacin**. Their **sodium** content is increased when boiled in sea water. Much of the potassium, calcium, phosphorus, chloride and niacin are lost in canned shrimps.

silicon A non-metallic element present in the human body in the cartilage and connective tissue. It is probably essential for humans, but this has not been established.

skate A large fatty fish of the ray family. It is considered to be the only fish that improves in flavour onces it becomes slightly 'high'. It provides **protein**, **fat** and small amounts of **potassium** and **magnesium**. It is generally eaten fried, which raises the energy value to 199 kcal/100 g, or poached, with an energy value of 96 kcal/100 g.

skin The soft and sensitive tissue covering the body. The condition of the skin is a good indicator of a person's general state of health. A healthy skin needs the full complement of essential **amino acids**, and – more importantly – of **essential fatty acids**. People on low-fat diets often develop skin disorders. The micronutrients that affect the skin most directly are **vitamin A** and **vitamin E** as well as **riboflavin**, **niacin**, **biotin**, **vitamin B₆**, **vitamin C**, **vitamin E**, **selenium** and **para-aminobenzoic acid**.

Deficiencies of one or several of these micronutrients may cause dryness, roughness, itching, scaliness, wrinkling, pale patches, pronounced stretch marks, slow healing of wounds and acne. Evening primrose oil, honey and infusions of cider vinegar or camomile are reported to have beneficial effects on a number of skin conditions. Skin diseases such as **eczema** and dermatitis can be caused by food allergy.

slimming   See APPENDIX I, LOSING AND GAINING WEIGHT.

smoked foods   Foods, usually meat, poultry, game, fish and cheese, that have been preserved by hanging them in smoke, traditionally that from a wood fire. The food is preserved by drying and by the action of a range of chemicals contained in the smoke. Smoking sometimes involves fairly high temperatures that deplete minerals and vitamins that are unstable at high temperatures, such as **thiamin**, **pantothenic acid** and **vitamin C**. Food to be smoked is often soaked in brine first to speed up the process. Such smoked food will have a high sodium content. Smoking reduces the water content so that – weight for weight – smoked foods have a higher energy value than their unsmoked equivalents.

smoking   The habit of smoking tobacco in cigarettes, cigars or pipes. The health risks of smoking cannot be overestimated. It is a major contributory factor to the most common causes of death in Britain, **coronary heart disease** and a number of forms of cancer. Cigarette smoke contains toxic lead, and a substance inhaled during smoking (acetaldehyde) depletes stores of **thiamin**, **vitamin B₆** and **vitamin C**. Smokers should supplement their diets with these vitamins, particularly vitamin C. Smoking has a very noticeable effect on the smoker's level of fitness. The build-up of tar in the lungs may cause respiratory difficulty and shortness of breath, and can lead to lung cancer. Smoking causes the arteries to 'fur up', therefore increasing the probability of cardiovascular diseases.

Smoking affects body weight, heavy smokers tend to weigh less for a given height than non-smokers, and many smokers observe an increase in body weight when they stop smoking. This may be partly due to the effect that smoking has on speeding up the rate of metabolism and also that smoking tends to deaden the senses of smell and taste so that less food is eaten. It is of course healthier to be a slightly over-weight non-smoker than a thin smoker. Non-smokers who live or work in close proximity to smokers are also at risk of developing many of the complaints associated with smoking.

soda water A soft drink made by artificially charging water with carbon dioxide to give it effervescence. The mineral content of soda water is usually negligible. Soda water should not be confused with carbonated **mineral waters**.

sodium An essential mineral found chiefly in the blood and the fluids that surround cells. The remainder is held inside cells and as part of the structure of bones. Together with **potassium**, sodium is a major factor in maintaining the balance of body fluid. It helps regulate the levels of acidity and alkalinity in the body, and it contributes to the functioning of muscles and nerves. It also stimulates the excretion of unwanted substances by the kidneys and, therefore, decreases the risk of kidney stones. The most common source of sodium is common **salt** (sodium chloride). In this form it is added to foods by manufacturers and in the home, in cooking and at the table. Foods that have a high sodium content are ham, bacon, sausages, cheese, seafood, smoked fish and kelp, as well as bread, other baked foods and breakfast cereals. There is no **RDA** for sodium, but a daily intake of 1–3.3 g is considered acceptable. The sodium content of the average diet is fairly high (about 2–4 g a day) and deficiency caused by the diet is unlikely.

Severe vomiting and diarrhoea or excessive sweating can dramatically reduce sodium levels resulting in dehydration, fatigue and apathy. High sodium intakes, which are far more common, have been linked with an increased susceptibility to **hypertension**, **stroke**, **heart disease** and stomach cancer. Whether a lower sodium intake can prevent hypertension is uncertain at present, but most authorities recommend a reduction. See also the introductory chapter, A BALANCED DIET.

sodium chloride The chemical name for **salt**.

soft drink Any of a number of non-alcoholic drinks, including squashes, cordials, fruit drinks and carbonated drinks. Soft drinks provide water and **sugars**, and have a variable, often high, energy value depending on the amount of sugar added. Although some contain fruit, the **vitamin C** content will not be significant unless it has been added by the manufacturer. The amounts of sucrose and fruit added to soft drinks are controlled by law, as are the energy values of low-calorie drinks. Many food additives are used in soft drinks, including preservatives, emulsifiers and flavouring.

sole A general name for several species of flat, white fish, including Dover sole and lemon sole. Sole contains **protein**, very little **fat** and has an energy value of 91 kcal/100 g (steamed). It also contains some **niacin**, **folic acid** and **pantothenic acid**. However, much of the niacin and some of the folic acid and pantothenic acid are lost if sole is steamed, and virtually all these micronutrients are lost if it is fried.

sorbet Water ice traditionally made from fruit juice or purée, sugar syrup and egg white. Sorbets usually have a high sugar content but little or no fat content. They, therefore, have a lower energy value than ice creams.

sorbitol A sugar alcohol present in apples, plums and cherries, and used as a **sweetener**, particularly in diabetic foods. Sorbitol has the same energy value as sucrose (394 kcal/100 g), but is considerably less sweet. It is metabolized slowly in the body to **fructose** and does not cause **insulin** reaction (see **blood glucose**). However, its use in diabetic diets is somewhat limited because of its **laxative** effect.

soup Consommés (clear soups), bisques (fish creams), vegetable purées, creams and broths are all types of soup. Almost any ingredient can be used in a soup, including meat, fish, poultry, vegetables and cereals, such as rice and barley and pulses, and dairy products such as milk and cheese. The nutritional values of soups vary enormously according to the ingredients but in general soups contain little **protein** and only small amounts of minerals and vitamins. Cream soups have higher **fat** contents and energy values, clear soups made from extracts or stock have very low energy values. Canned soup manufacturers follow a code of practice (standards set by the industry not the law) that ensures the amounts and quality of the ingredients. For example, a mixed vegetable soup should be made with a minimum of four different vegetables, or a green pea soup should be made from fresh or frozen peas. There are no such guidelines for dehydrated soups but – as with canned soups – all the ingredients must be listed on the label. Manufactured soups, particularly the instant dehydrated varieties, may contain food additives such as flavourings, colouring, emulsifiers, preservatives and **antioxidants**. Salt-free, additive-free and reduced-calorie soups are also available.

soya bean   A **pulse** or legume. The highly nutritious white-fleshed seed of an Asian bean plant. The soya bean provides **protein**, **fat**, mostly as **polyunsaturated fatty acids**, **starch**, **sugars** and **dietary fibre**, and has an energy value of 155 kcal/100 g (cooked beans). It is a good source of well-absorbed **iron**, which makes it a valuable part of vegetarian diets. Soya beans also contain **manganese**, **molybdenum**, **riboflavin**, **vitamin B_6**, **vitamin E** and **vitamin K**. It is one of the best plant sources of protein and is used as a meat substitute all over the world. It is also added to many manufactured foods to increase their protein content, e.g. sausages and beefburgers. The beans are eaten whole or sprouted, or processed into sauce, milk or curd. The oil is extracted and the residue is used for soya flour, **novel proteins** and cattle fodder. Uncooked soya beans contain **phytic acid** and **lectins**, and must be either well cooked or sprouted for some time for these to be destroyed. See also **soya bean oil**; **soya fibre**; **soya milk**; **soya sauce**; **tofu**.

soya bean oil   The vegetable oil extracted from the **soya bean**. Soya bean oil contains a high proportion of **polyunsaturated fatty acids**, particularly **linoleic acid**, and has an energy value of 899 kcal/100 g. It is a good source of **vitamin E** and **vitamin K** and is used commercially and domestically as a cooking oil. Soya bean oil is often used as the basis for margarines high in polyunsaturated fatty acids.

soya fibre The fibrous **soya bean** pulp left when the oil and soya milk have been extracted. It is an excellent source of **dietary fibre**, and contains a small proportion of the proteins and minerals associated with soya beans, but very little of the fat content that gives the soya bean its high energy value. It is used commercially to add bulk and texture to manufactured meat products, such as beefburgers, and meat substitutes, such as soya 'burgers'.

soya milk A milky substance obtained from crushed **soya beans**. Soya milk contains none of the dietary fibre in whole soya beans, but it does provide **protein, fat** (with a high proportion of **polyunsaturated fatty acids**), **starches** and **sugars**. It has an energy value of 39 kcal/100 g and also contains small amounts of **calcium**, **iron**, **riboflavin**, **vitamin B$_6$**, **vitamin E** and **vitamin K**. People allergic to cows' milk can usually tolerate soya milk and it makes a suitable alternative to cows' milk for **vegans**. It is also used to make **tofu**.

soya sauce A spicy, dark sauce made from fermented **soya beans** and wheat. It contains some

protein, **carbohydrate**, **calcium** and **potassium**, and has an energy value of 64 kcal/100 g. It is extremely high in **sodium**, because it contains added salt, and some brands contain **monosodium glutamate**.

spice   Any of a variety of seeds, stems or roots of certain aromatic plants that are used whole or ground to add flavour to food, e.g. **cumin**, **coriander**, **ginger**. They are used in such small quantities that their nutritional values are negligible.

spinach   A leafy green vegetable. It is a good source of **dietary fibre** and has an energy value of 30 kcal/100 g (boiled). Spinach contains more **protein** when compared with other vegetables. It is high in **sodium**, **potassium** and **carotene**, and contains some **copper**, **chlorides**, **manganese**, **riboflavin**, **vitamin C**, **vitamin E** and **vitamin K**. Although spinach has a high content of **iron** and **calcium**, the iron is poorly absorbed and the presence of **oxalic acid** prevents the absorption of calcium.

spirit, proof   A measure of the alcohol content of spirits and other alcoholic beverages. If a liquid were 100% proof it would contain 57% by volume or 49% by weight alcohol. 100% alcohol is, therefore, approximately 200% proof. As a general guideline, the percentage of alcohol in an alcoholic beverage is approximately half its spirit proof reading. The alcohol contents of beverages quoted in this book are measured as a percentage of alcohol per volume of the liquid.

spirits Distilled alcoholic liquors. Spirits are concentrated sources of **alcohol** with variable levels of sugar. They have high energy values, but are deficient in all other nutrients. See **brandy; gin; liqueur; vodka; whisky.**

spirulina A minute alga found in fresh water and alkaline lakes. Spirulina is almost self-supporting, taking energy from sunlight, carbon dioxide in the air and minerals from the water. It contains small amounts of protein, minerals and vitamins and is one of the few plant sources of **vitamin B$_{12}$** (it is, therefore a useful supplement for **vegans**).

sprat A small fatty fish of the herring family (immature sprats are also eaten, and are called brislings). Sprats provide **protein** and some **fat**, and they have an energy value of 441 kcal/100 g (fried). They also provide **calcium, phosphorus, iron** and a small amount of **niacin**. Sprats may be eaten fresh, usually fried, or smoked. Smoked sprats have a lower energy value of 225 kcal/100 g.

spring green Young mid-green leafy cabbages eaten before the heart has developed. Spring greens have a high water content and a correspondingly low energy value of 10 kcal/100 g. They provide very little **protein** and small amounts of

dietary fibre. Spring greens contain **carotene** and **riboflavin**, and some **manganese**, **zinc**, **vitamin C**, **folic acid** and **biotin**. Spring greens need to be boiled for some time to soften them, and this considerably reduces the vitamin C and folic acid contents.

spring onion A tiny, immature **onion** used to add flavour to salads. Spring onions contain rather more nutrients than mature onions. However, they are eaten in very small quantities and their nutritional values are virtually negligible.

sprouts Certain **pulses** or **seeds** moistened and allowed to sprout. Sprouts are good sources of **protein**, rich sources of **B complex vitamins** and also contain smaller amounts of **calcium**, **iron**, and **magnesium**. They are a very good source of **vitamin C**, particularly when eaten raw, but cooking and canning reduces the content. The pulses and seeds that are most commonly sprouted are **alfalfa**, **chickpeas**, **kidney beans**, **lentils**, **mung beans** and **soya beans**.

squash The large fruit of a marrow-like plant with a hard rind and pulpy flesh. Squashes have a high water content, a correspondingly low energy value of 25 kcal/100 g and contain only a very small amount of **protein**, and some **dietary fibre**. They also contain some **carotene**.

squash A soft drink that must by law contain 25% of fruit juice for undiluted citrus squash and

10% of fruit juice for non-citrus fruit squashes. Squashes must contain specified amounts of **sucrose** and **saccharin**, but these must be declared on the label.

squid A torpedo-shaped mollusc (see **shellfish**) with smooth, white flesh. Squid provides **protein**, very little **fat** and has an energy value of 66 kcal/100 g. It is rich in **iron** and also contains **sodium**, **potassium**, **calcium**, **phosphorus**, **sulphur**, **folic acid** and some **niacin**.

starch A **polysaccharide** composed of long chains of **glucose** units (molecules), and used as an energy store in most plants. Starch is broken down during digestion by enzymes into glucose, which is then absorbed into the bloodstream to supply energy. Uncooked starch is poorly digested. It is found in greatest quantities in bananas, bread, biscuits, cassava, corn, flour, oats, pearl barley, potatoes, semolina, sago, tapioca and yams. See also **modified starch**.

stabilizer A food additive used to prevent a mixture of substances that do not mix naturally from separating, such as fats and water. Stabilizers are often used by manufacturers together with emulsifiers in a variety of foods, including salad dressings, cakes, ice creams and margarines. **Edible gums**, **lecithin**, **agar**, **alginates**, chemically modified fats and chemically modified forms of **cellulose** are all permitted stabilizers.

steak A cut of lean meat usually from the rump or loin of an animal (most commonly beef, but also lamb or pork). There are several different cuts of steak, and their nutritional values vary. In general, they contain **protein** and variable amounts of **fat** with a high proportion of **saturated fatty acids**. The fat content can be reduced by buying lean cuts of meat, trimming off any visible fat and grilling rather than frying the steak. Steaks provide well-absorbed **iron** and **zinc**, as well as most of the **B complex vitamins**. None of these micronutrients are seriously depleted when steak is grilled. See also **stewing steak**.

steaming A method of cooking (usually vegetables or fish) by suspending the food over boiling water. Steaming has the advantage over boiling that fewer **micronutrients** are **leached** out during the cooking process. Only vitamins that are unstable at high temperatures, e.g. **pantothenic acid**, **thiamin** and **vitamin C**, will be seriously depleted by steaming.

stewing A method of cooking food in water or stock so that the temperature does not rise above simmering point (90°C). Stewed fruit does not take long to cook, but other foods, such as meat, take at least an hour. Stewed foods retain most of the vitamins and minerals of their raw ingredients, because they are served with the juices and because stewing involves moderate temperatures that do not destroy vitamins.

stewing steak A cut of beef (usually the brisket, chuck or skirt) that requires stewing for one or more hours to cook and tenderize it. It provides **protein** and **fat** with a high proportion of **saturated fatty acids**. The fat content can be reduced by removing any visible fat before cooking. It contains significant quantities of the same **micronutrients** as **steak**, but has a higher **sodium** content if salt is added to the stew.

stir frying A method of cooking that uses little or no **fat** and is carried out at very high temperatures for a short time. Only vitamins that are unstable at very high temperatures (e.g. **pantothenic acid**, **thiamin** and **vitamin C**) are seriously depleted by stir frying .

stock The juice obtained by boiling meat, fish or vegetables, or by adding water to stock cubes. Stock may be used to make soup or gravy, or it may be added to stews. Depending on the ingredients used, homemade stock may contain small amounts of **protein** and **fat**, and some of the vitamins that are **leached** into cooking water by boiling, e.g. **vitamin B$_6$, thiamin, riboflavin, niacin** and **pantothenic acid**.

stock cubes Ready-made stock preparations, usually prepared from meat, poultry or vegetable extracts. Stock cubes are added to soups and stews to give flavour. Their nutritional values vary according to the ingredients. In general, they have a very high **sodium** content and are likely to contain food additives.

stout A dark, sweet ale, highly flavoured with malt. Stout contains about 3% alcohol by volume, and has a higher sugar content than most beers. In extra stout, more of the **carbohydrate** has been turned to alcohol, and it contains about 4.5% alcohol by volume. Bottled stout has an energy value of 37 kcal/100 g (sixth of a pint).

strawberry The sweet, fleshy, red fruit of the strawberry plant. Strawberries contain **sugars**, a small amount of **dietary fibre** and have an energy value of 26 kcal/100 g. They are a good source of **vitamin C** and contain small amounts of **copper**, **folic acid** and **pantothenic acid**. Almost all the copper and some of the vitamin C, folic acid and pantothenic acid are lost in canned strawberries, but frozen strawberries retain almost all the vitamin C of fresh strawberries. Strawberries sweetened and canned have an energy value of 81 kcal/100 g.

stress A condition of physical or emotional strain. Stressful situations trigger the **adrenal gland** to release adrenaline, which accelerates the heart rate and increases the blood supply to the limbs and brain. In the wild, adrenaline is used to improve an animal's physical competence, but in modern man stressful situations are rarely accompanied by a need for physical exertion. If the release of adrenaline is not exploited by physical activity, the physiological changes it causes put considerable strain on the heart and give rise to the 'jittery' feeling many people experience at times of stress. Prolonged or repeated periods of stress may cause loss of appetite, insomnia and irritability, and may give rise to a number of physiological complaints such as gastric ulcers. Stress may also cause people to increase the amount they smoke and drink.

The harmful effects of stress and the symptoms themselves may be reduced by an increased intake of **thiamin**, **niacin**, **vitamin B$_6$**, **vitamin C** and **inositol**. Regular exercise and a healthy diet will ensure that the heart is in peak condition to cope with the strain of excessive adrenal activity. Some herbal infusions (e.g. **camomile**, **passion flower**, **rosemary** and **valerian**) are attributed with sedative qualities, and **royal jelly** is reported to alleviate the symptoms of stress in many people.

string bean See **runner bean**.

stroke A disease that affects the blood vessels in the brain. It may involve brain haemorrhages and obstructions, such as a clot in a brain artery. Such an obstruction may cut off of the blood supply to parts of the brain, resulting in brain damage. Those most at risk of having a stroke are people who are prone to **hypertension**, **atherosclerosis** or **obesity**. To minimize the risks of a stroke, intakes of **salt**, **fat** and particularly **saturated fatty acids**

and **alcohol** should be moderated, body weight should be controlled and some form of exercise should be taken regularly.

sucrose (common name **sugar**) A **carbohydrate**, or **disaccharide** of **glucose** and **fructose**. It occurs naturally in beet and cane sugar, from which it is commercially refined, and in smaller amounts in fruit and some root vegetables. It is available in many forms in various stages of refinement: white sugars (e.g. caster, granulated and icing sugar) are the most refined; brown sugars (e.g. demerara and muscovado) are less refined; sugars that are described as raw (e.g. raw cane sugar) are the least refined. Sugar is consumed in foods such as preserves, cordials, confectionary, cakes and biscuits. It is used commercially as a **sweetener** and a preservative.

Sucrose is broken down by enzymes in the digestive tract to its constituent monosaccharides, glucose and fructose, which are absorbed and carried in the blood to the liver and used for energy supply. Sucrose is virtually 100% **carbohydrate** and has an energy value of 394 kcal/100 g, but no other nutritional value. Sugar encourages the growth of bacteria that cause **dental caries** and may cause yeasts in the body to multiply so rapidly that yeast infections develop. The diet of many people would benefit from a reduction in sugar consumption. See also the introductory chapter, A BALANCED DIET.

suet A tough, dry, waxy deposit of fat found

around certain organs of animals, particularly the kidneys of beef and mutton. Suet fat is high in **saturated fatty acids** and has a high energy value of 826 kcal/100 g, but contains negligible **micronutrients**.

sugar   See **sucrose**.

sugars   Simple **carbohydrates** (monosaccharides and disaccharides) present in food and including **sucrose**, **glucose**, **fructose**, **maltose** and **lactose**. They are all sweet-tasting and have the same energy value of 394 kcal/100 g.

sulphur   A non-metallic mineral that, along with potassium, is the third most common mineral in the body (after calcium and phosphorus). It is present in the essential **amino acid** methionine, and the non-essential amino acid cysteine, and is a component of **biotin** and **thiamin**. Apart from cysteine, these substances cannot be synthesized by the body, so they must be supplied by the diet. In order to ensure a good intake of the essential amino acids that contain sulphur, the diet should contain **protein** or a variety of sources of protein. The amino acids and vitamins that contain sulphur are responsible for maintaining healthy hair, nails and skin, for promoting mental activity and the secretion of bile. A deficiency of these sulphur-related compounds causes dry hair and skin, cracking nails and an increased susceptibility to **arthritis**.

sultana   A dried white grape (a dried black grape is called a raisin). Sultanas are a rich source of **sugars** (mostly **glucose** and **fructose**), contain some **dietary fibre** and have an energy value of 250 kcal/100 g. They provide **potassium** and **iron**, and smaller amounts of other minerals and vitamins.

sunflower seeds   The small, highly nutritious seeds of the sunflower, with tough black and white striped skin and a smooth, oily stone-coloured and pleasantly flavoured kernel. Sunflower seeds provide an exceptionally good source of **protein** for a plant source, and have a high **polyunsaturated fatty acid** content (including a high percentage of **linoleic acid**). They contain some **sugars** and **starch**, and have an energy value of 524 kcal/100 g. Sunflower seeds are a good source of **vitamin E**, and they provide **vitamin A**, **B complex vitamins**, **vitamin D**, **iron**, **potassium**, **phosphorus**, **magnesium**, **manganese**, **copper** and **calcium**.

sunflower oil   The vegetable oil extracted from sunflower seeds. Sunflower oil is used for cooking and dressings. It has a high **polyunsaturated fatty acid** content (including a high percentage of **linoleic acid**), is a good source of **vitamin E** and has an energy value of 899 kcal/100 g.

supplement   A concentrated source of **nutrients** and **micronutrients**. Supplements are usually available as dry tablets, capsules or tonics and may be synthesized or naturally occurring substances. They may contain concentrates of one, several or all the vitamins and minerals. They may be used by people whose diet is likely to be deficient in certain micronutrients, and by those who have increased requirements for some or all micronutrients (e.g. growing children, the elderly, the sick and the convalescent, women who are pregnant, lactating or menstruating, athletes and slimmers). Some people take supplements as an 'insurance' against the possible ill-effects of a poor diet, the contraceptive pill, alcohol, smoking and stress. Very large doses (megadoses) of vitamins and minerals sometimes form part of the treatment of certain illnesses and diseases, but such therapy is controversial. See **megavitamin therapy**.

swede The bulbous, edible root of a plant of Eurasian origin, with pulpy, orange flesh that is eaten as a vegetable. Swedes have a high water content and contain some **sugars**, no starch and only small amounts of **protein**, **dietary fibre** (including **pectin**), **B complex vitamins** and **vitamin C**. They have an energy value of 18 kcal/100 g.

sweetcorn The tender, sweet-tasting, yellow kernels of unripe **maize**. Sweetcorn is available fresh on the cob (in which case it needs to be boiled before it is eaten) or pre-cooked and canned. It contains **starch,** some **protein** and **dietary fibre**, a small amount of **sugars** and some **magnesium**, **copper**, **zinc**, **manganese**, **molybdenum**, **phosphorus**, **thiamin**, **niacin** and **vitamin E**. Much of the magnesium, copper, zinc and thiamin and some of the niacin and vitamin E are lost in canned sweetcorn. Boiled corn on the cob has an energy value of 123 kcal/100 g and canned sweetcorn has a value of 76 kcal/100 g.

sweetener   A substance that stimulates the sweet-sensitive taste buds of the tongue. Sweeteners include naturally occurring **sugars**, such as **glucose** and **sucrose**. The term is also applied to sugar-related compounds called 'bulk' sweeteners. These include **sorbitol** and **glucose syrup**, which have the same energy values as sugars (394 kcal/100 mg). Like sugars, they add to the volume of the food in which they are used. There are also artificial sweetening agents, such as **saccharin** and **aspartame**, which are known as 'intense' sweeteners. These have different chemical structures to sugars, and are up to 600 times as sweet, weight for weight. They are used in only very small quantities and do not add to the bulk of foods. They have virtually no energy value and are used in the manufacture of reduced-calorie foods and drinks. They are also available as table-top sweeteners.

sweet peppers   See **peppers**.

sweet potato   The large, edible root of a tropical twining plant with yellow flesh, eaten as a vegetable. Sweet potatoes contain **starch**, **sugars**, some **dietary fibre** and a small amount of **protein** and they have an energy value of 85 kcal/100 g (boiled). They also contain **potassium**, **phosphorus**, **carotene**, **thiamin**, **niacin** and **vitamin E**, and small amounts of **vitamin A** and **vitamin C**. Only some of the vitamin C content is lost when sweet potatoes are boiled.

syrup A concentrated solution of different **sugars**. Maple syrup is a natural extract of the maple tree. Other syrups – which include **molasses**, **treacle** and golden syrup – are by-products obtained during the refining of sugar crystals. Syrups are virtually pure sugars and have a high energy value. They possess the same undesirable properties as **sucrose**. Except for molasses, most syrups have little or no nutritional value.

table salt See **salt**.

tahini A smooth, oily paste made from crushed **sesame seeds**. The husks of the seeds may be included in the paste, making it dark and grainy, with a more bitter taste. It is high in **polyunsaturated fatty acids** (including **linoleic acid**) and contains some **protein** and **dietary fibre** (if the husks are included). Because of the high fat content it has a high energy value of 607 kcal/100 g. Like sesame seeds it contains **calcium**, **magnesium** and **iron**, but because of the presence of **phytic acid**, which forms insoluble salts with these minerals, little is available for absorption into the bloodstream. Tahini is also rich in **potassium**, which is well absorbed.

tangerine A small citrus fruit of Asian origin, with bright orange, characteristically loose rind and sweet, spicy, orange flesh in crescent-shaped segments, with very few seeds. Tangerines are related to mandarins and satsumas, and are thought to have been crossed with a variety of orange to obtain clementines. They contain some **sugars** and **dietary fibre** and provide useful amounts of **vitamin C**, and have an energy value of 34 kcal/100 g. Canned tangerines contain more sugar and less vitamin C than fresh ones, and have an energy value of 56 kcal/100 g.

tannins A group of chemicals, called polyphenols, that have astringent properties and are present in some plants such as tea. Tannins are used to clarify beer and wines and they may contribute unfavourably to their flavour. As red wine ages it becomes less astringent because the tannins undergo chemical changes. Tannins are responsible for the bitter taste left in the mouth by a strong cup of tea. They act as antinutrients, i.e. they inhibit the **absorption** of nutrients, particularly iron.

tapioca Grainy **starch** obtained from the root of the cassava plant. Tapioca is available as pellets, flakes, granules or flour, and it is used commercially and domestically in puddings and as a thickening agent. It contains 95% starch and, therefore, has a high energy value of 359 kcal/100 g. It does not contain significant quantities of any

micronutrients. The lack of nutritional content is overcome when it is cooked with milk.

taramasalata A smooth, characteristically pink paste made with smoked cod's **roe**, olive oil and breadcrumbs. It has a high **fat** content, contains a little **protein** and has an energy value of 482 kcal/100 g. Taramasalata usually contains added salt and, therefore, has a high **sodium** content. It may also contain artificial colouring, flavouring and preservatives.

tarragon The small, toothed leaves of an aromatic, perennial plant that are used fresh or dried, chopped or powdered, as a herb. Tarragon is consumed in such small quantities that its nutritional properties are negligible. Infusions of tarragon are believed to relieve insomnia and to have a number of beneficial effects on the digestive tract, such as promoting the appetite and stimulating the secretion of digestive juices.

tartrazine A synthetic yellow food colouring (E102) widely used in many foods, drugs and drinks, including fruit squashes, instant puddings, custard powder and sweets. Of all food additives, tartrazine appears to be the most reactive, causing migraine, nettle rash, runny nose, asthma and **hyperactivity** in children. Between 3 in 10 000 and 1 in 1000 people are currently thought to be sensitive to tartrazine.

tea An infusion of dried, fermented leaves of one or several varieties of evergreen tropical or sub-tropical shrub. Tea commonly originates from India, Sri Lanka, Kenya and China. Indian, Sri Lankan and Kenyan tea is usually strong and very dark. China tea is generally served weaker and has a more aromatic taste. It may contain flavourings, such as bergamot in Earl Grey tea. Tea is drunk hot or chilled, with or without lemon or milk and/or sugar, and tea itself has no energy value. It contains stimulants, **caffeine** and theophylline (stronger and more harmful than caffeine) and **tannins**. It contains the trace elements **manganese** and **fluoride**, and small amounts of **riboflavin** and **niacin**. Large quantities of tea interfere with the absorption of **iron**, and if tea is drunk with a meal it can significantly reduce the absorption of iron from the food.

Many teas named after fruits or flowers (e.g. **jasmine tea**) are made with traditional tea to which varying amounts of fruits or flowers have been added. They have comparable levels of caffeine, theophylline and tannins as ordinary tea. **Herb teas** and true infusions of fruits and flowers do not contain these substances and some of them are believed to have medicinal properties.

tooth Strong bone-like structure covered in natural enamel and set in the jaw for biting and chewing food. Good supplies of **vitamin D, calcium, magnesium, phosphorus, fluorine** and **molybdenum** are needed to maintain strong, healthy teeth. See also **dental caries**.

textured vegetable protein The textured or

extruded type of **novel protein** made from **soya flour** that has a fibrous texture similar to meat. It is relatively cheap to manufacture and is used by caterers and food manufacturers to extend the meat in products such as meat pies, stews, curries and sausages. It cannot be used to replace the legal minimum meat content in meat products, but it can be used in addition if declared on the label. It contains as much, or more, **protein** as meat, but of an inferior quality because it contains less of the essential **amino acid** methionine. It is also lacking in **vitamins B₁, B₂, and B₁₂**. As it contains **phytic acid**, the **zinc** and **iron** are less readily available to the body. It is low in **fat** but high in **sugars** and **starch**. There are no compositional standards set by the Ministry of Agriculture, Fisheries and Food for textured vegetable protein, but many manufacturers improve the quality by adding the amino acid, methionine, and vitamins B₁, B₂, B₁₂.

thiamin (also called **vitamin B₁**) One of the **B complex vitamins**, essential for growth and metabolism, particularly concerned with the release of energy from **glucose**. Good sources of thiamin include wholegrain cereals, pork, bacon, ham, offal, nuts and pulses. It can also be obtained from brewer's yeast, yeast, yeast extract and wheat germ. Thiamin is very easily destroyed in the cooking and preparation of food, even thawing when it is **leached** into the drip. The body is less well able to absorb thiamin in the presence of alcohol, caffeine, antibiotics and the contraceptive pill. Thiamin requirements are closely related to **carbohydrate** intake. The UK **RDAs** are based on an average requirement of 0.4 mg per 1000 kcal. Deficiency symptoms include nausea, vomiting, loss of weight, lack of sleep and depression. Mental confusion, loss of feeling and muscle weakness in the limbs develop as the deficiency disease progresses towards **berberi**.

tin A metal that is present in the body and is possibly an essential **trace element**. Canned foods and foods wrapped in tin foil contain more tin than fresh foods. Tin is used in the treatment of a number of skin complaints, including acne and boils.

tocopherol See **vitamin E**.

tofu A smooth, bland curd made from the yellow **soya bean** and available either in a firm or silken junket-like form. Tofu is a good source of **protein**, particularly for vegetarians and **vegans**. It is low in **fat** and therefore has a low energy value of 70 kcal/per 100 g, and is a rich source of **calcium**. Because of its bland flavour it can be readily combined with other ingredients.

tomato The fleshy, red, many-seeded fruit of the tomato plant, a member of the nightshade family. Tomatoes have a high water content and therefore a low energy value of 14 kcal/per 100 g. They supply appreciable amounts of **carotene** and **vitamin C**, but some of the vitamin C is lost in canned tomatoes.

Tomato juice has the lowest energy value of all fruit juices, 16 kcal/per 100 g. Some of the vitamin C in a whole fresh tomato is lost in the manufacture of tomato juice. Tomato juice may include added salt, which increases the **sodium** content.

tomato juice See **tomato**.

tongue The highly sensitive and mobile organ in the mouth. The tongue is used to manipulate food in the mouth and it participates in the sense of taste. Deficiencies of **riboflavin**, **vitamin B₆** and **folic acid** may cause inflammations of the tongue, which can be corrected by increasing the intake of these vitamins, either in the diet or in supplements. If the symptoms persist, medical advice should be sought. See also **ulcers**.

tongue (offal) The tongues of lamb, ox, calves and pigs that are eaten as meat. Tongue contains **protein** and well-absorbed **iron**. It is high in **fat**, with a high proportion of **saturated fatty acids** and therefore has a high energy value of 290 kcal/100 g. Tongue is available pickled, which has a very high salt and, therefore, **sodium** content, and it also contains **nitrate** and **nitrite**.

tonic water An artificially carbonated mixer that traditionally contains quinine and has a delicate orange flavour. Tonic water contains some **sugars** and has an energy value of 25 kcal/100 ml. Low-calorie tonic water with artificial sweeteners is also available. Quinine is used as a general tonic and to alleviate pain and fever (especially in malaria). Tonic water may contain artificial colourings and flavourings.

tooth decay   See **dental caries**.

trace elements   **Minerals** necessary to the body in much smaller amounts than the major or bulk minerals. The trace elements are **cobalt**, **copper**, **chromium**, **fluorine**, **iodine**, **iron**, **manganese**, **molybdenum**, **selenium**, vanadium and **zinc**. The **RDA** of all the trace elements is less than 100 mg. In most cases, their importance has been established more recently than that of the bulk minerals and is perhaps not yet fully understood. Excess amounts are toxic and there is often a small difference between the amount needed for health and the amount that is toxic. Too much of one trace element can cause a deficiency of another. Eating a moderate amount of a wide variety of foods reduces the risk of obtaining too much or too little.

treacle   The name given either to black treacle or to golden syrup. Black treacle is a true **syrup**, a by-product obtained during the refining of sugar crystals. It is dark and viscous because it has been subjected to high temperatures, and is very concentrated. Golden syrup is a honey-coloured fluid made by evaporating the water from cane sugar juice. Both are high in **sugars** and have energy values of 257 kcal/100 g (black treacle) and 298 kcal/100 g (golden syrup). Black treacle contains slightly more **protein** than golden syrup. It has a high **potassium** content and provides useful amounts of **calcium**, **magnesium**, and **iron**. Both possess the undesirable properties of sugar.

triglyceride The chemical name for most common forms of **fat** in food. Each molecule of triglyceride is made up of one molecule of **glycerol** and three (tri-) **fatty acids**.

tripe The stomach lining of sheep or ox which is eaten as offal. The nutritional values of different kinds of tripe vary, but in general it contains a small amount of **protein** and some **fat**, with a high content of **saturated fatty acids**. It is nutritionally poor and does not contain significant amounts of any **micronutrients**, although when cooked with milk (as it usually is) the nutrient content is increased. It has a distinctive taste, not universally enjoyed, and indeed most tripe is used in the manufacture of pet foods.

trout A general name for several varieties (brown or river trout, rainbow trout and sea trout) of fatty freshwater or saltwater fish of the salmon family. Trout contains **protein** and, although classed as a fatty fish, little **fat**. It has an energy value of 135 kcal/100 g (steamed trout) and contains only negligible amounts of **micronutrients**, which are further lowered when it is cooked. Sea trout contains more **sodium** than brown or rainbow trout.

tuber A fleshy, usually bulbous root or underground stem of a plant, eaten as a vegetable. Tubers are a plant's food store and they tend to be higher in **carbohydrate** (either as starch or sugars) than other vegetables. Some tubers contain aromatic, volatile oils and are valued for these properties, e.g. **ginger**, **ginseng**, **horseradish** and **turmeric**. See **beetroot**; **carrot**; **cassava**; **celeriac**; **Jerusalem artichoke**; **parsnip**; **potato**; **swede**; **sweet potato**; **turnip**; **yam**.

tuna A large warm-water fatty fish with pink, meaty flesh. Tuna is served fresh, or canned in vegetable oil or brine. It contains **protein** and some **fat**, with a high proportion of **polyunsaturated fatty acids**. It provides appreciable amounts of **vitamin D**, **vitamin E** and **vitamin B$_6$**. Tuna canned in vegetable oil has a high fat content and a correspondingly high energy value of 293 kcal/ 100 g, tuna canned in brine has an energy value of 107 kcal/100 g and fresh tuna an energy value of 157 kcal/100 g. Tuna canned in brine has a higher **sodium** content than fresh tuna or tuna canned in oil.

turkey A domestic fowl of North American origin, and its meat. Turkey contains **protein** and is low in **fat**, and therefore has a low energy value of 140 kcal/100 g of roast turkey meat. It supplies well-absorbed **iron** and **zinc** (more in dark meat than white meat).

turmeric The aromatic, yellow-coloured underground stem of a tropical Asian plant, powdered and used to give flavour and colour to food. Turmeric is consumed in such small quantities that its nutritional value is negligible.

turnip The leaves (turnip tops) and white or yellowish roots of a Mediterranean plant, eaten as a vegetable. Turnips (the roots) have a high water content and contain some **sugars** and **dietary fibre** (including **pectins**). They do not contain significant quantities of any **micronutrients** and have a low energy value of 14 kcal/100 g (boiled turnips). The leaves of turnips are a good source of **vitamin A**, **vitamin C**, **vitamin E**, **riboflavin** and **folic acid**. They have an energy value of 11 kcal/100 g (boiled turnip leaves).

tyramine A derivative of the **amino acid** tyrosine that is found in some meat and yeast extracts, cheese, chocolate and some wines. These foods should be avoided when certain tranquilizers (monoamine oxidase inhibitors) are being taken as they react with tyramine and cause a severe rise in blood pressure. In the absence of these drugs, the body can detoxify tyramine with an enzyme called monoamine oxidase.

ugli fruit A large citrus fruit with loose, wrinkled, bumpy greenish-yellow skin and juicy, yellow flesh in crescent-shaped segments. The ugli fruit originated in the West Indies and was obtained by crossing oranges, grapefruits and tangerines. It provides some **sugars**, **dietary fibre** and **vitamin C** and an energy value of 55 kcal/100 g.

UHT   See **ultra heat treated**.

ulcer   A disintegration of the surface of the mucous membrane, causing one or more highly sensitive sores in the mouth or any other part of the digestive tract. Ulcers in the mouth and on the tongue (apthous ulcers) tend to be very small and to heal quickly. Peptic ulcers, which occur in other parts of the digestive tract (most commonly the duodenum, sometimes the stomach and rarely the oesophagus), are a common and painful complaint, more prevalent in men than women. The underlying cause is unknown, but – especially in the case of duodenal ulcers – worry, stress and overwork are important predisposing factors. People with a susceptibility to developing ulcers should avoid smoking, caffeine, too much alcohol, highly spiced food and fried food. Infusions of **verbena** may temporarily soothe ulcers. People suffering from ulcers or suspected ulcers should seek medical advice.

ultra heat treated (UHT)   A method of sterilizing foods, usually milk, using very high temperatures. Ultra heat treatment is used to extend the shelf life of foods. It involves higher temperatures (130°)

than **pasteurization**, but over a shorter period (two seconds). Nutrient losses are similar to those that occur during pasteurization (25% loss of **vitamin C** and 10% loss of **thiamin**, **vitamin B₆**, **folic acid** and **vitamin B₁₂**), but UHT milk can be stored for long periods and up to 50% loss of vitamin B₆ and vitamin B₁₂ will have occurred after three months of storage. Once the sealed container is opened, UHT milk is as perishable as pasteurized milk.

urticaria The formation of red or whitish, itchy raised patches on any part of the skin, occasionally swelling of the lips, face, tongue and more rarely mouth and throat. It is a common symptom of food allergy, although there are other non-food related causes. The foods most likely to cause urticaria are nuts, fish and eggs. Additives, such as colours and preservatives, may also provoke such a reaction.

vanilla The dark aromatic pod of certain varieties of tropical climbing orchid, used for flavouring food. The pod may be ground up and used in food, or – more usually – soaked (e.g. in milk) to permeate the liquid with its flavour. The nutritional value of vanilla is negligible, because it is consumed in such small quantities. Vanilla essence is made by extracting the **essential oil** that gives the pod its distinctive flavour. This essence and foods labelled 'vanilla flavour' may also contain artificial flavouring and colourings.

veal The flesh of the young calf (not more than

three months) that has been fed exclusively on milk or other foods low in iron in order to keep the flesh white. Veal contains **protein**, a level of **fat** and **saturated fatty acids** similar to lean **beef** and has an energy value of 230 kcal/100 g (roast meat). It is about half the **iron** content of beef, and provides useful amounts of **phosphorus** and **niacin**, and smaller amounts of **riboflavin**, **pyridoxine** and **thiamin**.

vegan A person who consumes no animal products at all and whose diet is totally vegetable and cereal based. See APPENDIX II, VEGETARIAN, VEGAN AND MACROBIOTIC DIETS.

vegetable juice The juice of one of several crushed or pulped vegetables. The nutritional values depend on the vegetables that are used, but juices contain none of the **dietary fibre** that may be present in the whole vegetables from which they are derived. In general, vegetable juices have low energy values, of the order of 14 kcal/100 g. They may contain added salt and, therefore, have high **sodium** contents.

vegetable oil Any oil extracted from the seeds or nuts of plants, either by crushing or, more commonly, by using solvents. Vegetable oils are 99.9% fat and, therefore, have very high energy values of 899 kcal/100 g. Most vegetable oils have a higher content of **polyunsaturated fatty acids** and a lower content of **saturated fatty acids**, compared with animal fats. Such fatty acid compositions have the beneficial effect of lowering blood **cholesterol** levels. Corn oil, safflower seed oil, soya bean oil, walnut and sunflower oil are high in polyunsaturated fatty acids, including **linoleic acid**. Olive oil, rape-seed oil, groundnut and wheat germ oil contain more mono-unsaturated fatty acids and probably have a neutral effect on blood cholesterol levels. Coconut oil and palm oil are very low in polyunsaturated fatty acids and high in saturated fatty acids (especially palm oil). In general, vegetable oils are good sources of **vitamin E**, but contain no other vitamins and minerals (except red palm oil, which contains **carotene**).

vegetables The edible leaves, fruit, roots, flowers or stalks of plants. Vegetables may be eaten raw (in some cases) or cooked, and are available fresh, frozen, canned or dried (in some cases). Vegetables have low energy values because of their high water contents. However, root vegetables (see **tubers**) contain more **starch** and less water than non-root vegetables and consequently have higher energy values. For example, boiled cabbage has an energy value of 7 kcal/100 g and boiled carrots 19 kcal/100 g. The **carbohydrate** content of vegetables occurs as **sugars**, starch and **dietary fibre** in varying amounts, depending on the part of the plant. In general, vegetables provide very little **protein** (see **pulses** for good plant sources of protein) or **fat** (see **vegetable oils** for plant sources of fat). The amounts of vitamins and minerals they contain varies, but most vegetables (especially dark green, leafy vegetables) are important sources of **folic acid**, **riboflavin**, **vitamin A** (in the form of **carotene**) and **vitamin C**.

Vitamin C and folic acid are easily destroyed by poor cooking practices. In order to minimize losses, vegetables should be cooked in a very small amount of water for the shortest possible time. Steaming or microwave cooking conserve the greatest proportion of vitamins. Freezing vegetables does not affect the vitamin content, but vitamin C and folic acid contents gradually decline in storage. Further losses can occur if the manufacturers' cooking instructions are not followed. Canned vegetables are sterilized by heat, which causes losses of vitamin C, folic acid and thiamin. Dehydrating vegetables causes vitamin C losses. The use in dehydration processes of sulphur dioxide (a preservative declared on the label) preserves vitamin C but destroys thiamin. See **asparagus; aubergine; avocado pear; bamboo shoot; broccoli; Brussels sprout; cabbage; cauliflower; celery; chicory; Chinese leaf; courgette; cucumber; dahls; endive; fennel; globe artichoke; kale; kelp; lettuce; marrow; mushroom; onion; pumpkin; salsify; seakale; shallot; spinach; spring green; spring onion; squash; sweet potato; sweetcorn; tomato; watercress**.

vegetarian A person who excludes meat, poultry and fish from their diet, but not dairy products or, usually, eggs. See APPENDIX II, VEGETARIAN,

VEGAN AND MACROBIOTIC DIETS.

venison The flesh of deer, usually served roasted or in stews. Venison provides **protein**, is low in **fat** and has an energy value of 198 kcal/100 g (roast meat). It is a rich source of **iron** and also contains useful amounts of **thiamin**.

verbena The leaves of a red, white or purple-flowered plant originally from the Americas. Verbena leaves (usually dried) are used whole or crushed to make an infusion which is popular, particularly in France, as an evening drink because it acts as a mild sedative. It has beneficial effects on the digestive tract (including soothing ulcers and indigestion) and the respiratory tract (it is an expectorant).

vinegar A sharp-tasting, acid liquid usually obtained as a by-product of malted barley wine, cider or spirits. Vinegar is used for flavouring foods and as a preservative in pickled foods (malt vinegar has a less pleasant flavour than cider or other vinegars and it is more commonly used for pickling than these, which are better suited for adding flavour and making salad dressings). The main ingredient of vinegar is **acetic acid**. It has virtually no energy value, and contains only traces of **B complex vitamins** and **minerals**. The food additive caramel is often used to colour vinegar brown. See also **cider vinegar**; **wine vinegar**.

vitamin Any one of a number of organic substances needed by the body in very small amounts to help growth, metabolism and general health. The word vitamin is derived from the Latin *vita* (life) and *amine* (a chemical group once believed to be a part of all vitamins). There are some 20 vitamins, most of which cannot be synthesized by the body, and they must, therefore, be obtained from the diet. Each vitamin performs one or several functions within the body. An **RDA** (recommended daily amount) for most vitamins has been established to act as a guideline to requirements. However, this figure varies according to age, sex and occupation, and may be affected by illness, pregnancy, lactation and times of stress or rigorous activity.

Different foods contain different amounts of vitamins, and some of their vitamin content may be depleted by cooking or food processing. If the body does not absorb sufficient quantities of any or all the vitamins, it displays deficiency symptoms. It is also possible to consume too much of some vitamins and they can reach toxic levels in the body. The vitamins that are more likely to reach toxic levels are those that are fat-soluble (**vitamin A**, **vitamin D**, **vitamin E** and **vitamin K**). The body cannot eliminate excesses but stores them in the body. The other vitamins (**vitamin C** and the **B complex vitamins**) are water soluble and excesses can be eliminated in the urine. In a well-balanced diet there should be no danger of vitamin deficiency or toxicity. For information on the functions, food sources, stability, RDA and deficiency and toxicity symptoms of the individual vitamins, see separate entries.

vitamin A (also called **retinol**)   A vitamin essential for growth and for the maintainence of healthy skin and mucous membranes in the eyes, ears, nose, throat, lungs and bladder. Vitamin A is a component of the photosensitive pigment in the eye which is responsible for perceiving dim and red or green light (it is, therefore, important to good night vision and, in good light, to the differentiation of colours). Liver is the richest source of retinol; other good sources are kidney, eggs, dairy products and margarine. Fish liver oils, such as cod liver oil, are rich in retinol and may be used as supplements. It can also be derived from its precursor **carotene**. It is fairly stable to heat, but it is sensitive to light and oxygen, and is destroyed by rancid fats. The adult **RDA** for vitamin A is 750 µg. A deficiency first causes sore, itchy eyes and poor, dry skin. Vision at night becomes difficult leading to night blindness. The corneas of the eyes become damaged because of lack of secretions and eventually there is permanent blindness. Vitamin A deficiency is rare in Western countries, but it is a major cause of blindness in many countries of the Third World. Vitamin A is stored in the liver, and if it is consumed in excessive quantities (more than 10 times the RDA) it may reach toxic levels, which cause headaches, loss of appetite and poor skin and hair condition.

vitamin B₁   See **thiamin**.

vitamin B₂ See **riboflavin**.

vitamin B₃ See **niacin**.

vitamin B₄, B₇, B₉, B₁₀, B₁₁, B₁₄, B₁₆ These are vitamins no longer considered essential to man.

vitamin B₅ See **pantothenic acid**.

vitamin B₆ (also called **pyridoxine**) One of the B complex vitamins. Vitamin B₆ is essential for growth and is a key factor in the formation of new **proteins**. It performs a number of other important functions in the body, including: releasing the stores of energy in the liver, possibly converting **linoleic acid** into other essential **fatty acids**, maintaining the correct balance of **sodium** and **potassium**, and contributing to the forming of antibodies and red blood cells. It is found in meats, cheese, liver, fish, wholegrain cereals and wholemeal bread, many vegetables, nuts, bananas, avocado pears and brewer's yeast. It is lost by **leaching** into cooking water and during thawing, and is depleted by the contraceptive pill. There is no UK **RDA**, but the US RDA is 2.2 mg for men and 2.0 mg for women. No adult disease has been specifically attributed to lack of pyridoxine in the diet, but deficiencies may occur if an antagonistic drug is taken in combination with a poor intake. Symptoms include the appearance of ridges on nails, sensitivity to sunlight, cracking of the lips, numbness of hands and feet, skin disorders and convulsions (particularly in young children).

vitamin B₁₂ (also called cobalamin) One of the **B complex vitamins**. Vitamin B_{12} is vital for growth and for the correct formation of red blood cells. It is also important to the maintenance of a healthy nervous system because it helps form the fatty sheath around nerves. Liver is a particularly rich source of vitamin B_{12}, but all animal foods supply it: offal, fatty fish, shellfish, meat, cheese, white fish, eggs and milk. It is almost entirely absent from plants, and **vegans** can become deficient unless they eat foods supplemented with vitamin B_{12} (SEE APPENDIX II, VEGETARIAN, VEGAN AND MACROBIOTIC DIETS). Vitamin B_{12} is fairly stable to heat, but like other B complex vitamins **leaches** out of foods into the cooking water. Up to half can be lost in cooking meat. There is no UK **RDA**, but a daily intake of 2 µg is generally considered adequate. A deficiency causes a form of **anaemia** called pernicious anaemia.

vitamin B₁₅ See **pangamic acid**.

vitamin B₁₇ See **laetrile**.

vitamin C (also called ascorbic acid) A vitamin essential for growth and vital for the formation of collagen (a protein necessary to healthy bones, teeth, skin, gums, blood capillaries and all connective tissue); as such, it plays an important role in the healing of wounds and of fractures. Vitamin C increases the **absorption** of **calcium** and **iron**, and helps excrete toxic minerals such as lead, copper and mercury. The best sources of vitamin C are blackcurrants, broccoli, green peppers, strawberries, cabbage, fresh citrus fruits, potatoes, peas, parsley and watercress. It is the least stable vitamin and much of it is lost during the preparation and cooking of food. It is destroyed by heat and alkalinity and is lost through **leaching** in all cooking processes. To maintain their vitamin C content, foods should be cooked in very little water for a minimum of time and served immediately. The UK adult RDA is 30 mg but the US RDA is twice that amount. Smokers have greater requirements for vitamin C than normal.

Vitamin C deficiency is the cause of the disease **scurvy**, which increases susceptibility to infections, especially colds, as well as causing general tiredness and loss of appetite. Over a prolonged period, it can cause haemorrhages, loss of teeth and weakening of bones, and – ultimately – sudden death from internal haemorrhage. Large doses of vitamin C taken at the onset of a cold can minimize the symptoms, but regular dosing does not prevent a cold. Very large doses of vitamin C should be avoided by people who are susceptible to kidney stones, because it is converted to **oxalic acid** within the body.

vitamin D   A vitamin essential for growth, for the **absorption** of calcium from food and for the hardening of bones with **calcium** and **phosphorus**. Both these elements are vital to healthy teeth as well as bones. It also assists in maintaining a healthy nervous system and sound circulation. It is found in cod liver oil or other fish liver oils, herring, fatty fish, margarine and eggs. Vitamin D is sometimes called the 'sunshine vitamin' because when the skin is exposed to sunlight, the ultra-violet rays convert a derivative of **cholesterol** in the skin into vitamin D. This process is much reduced in Asian skin. However, West Indians are no more susceptible than white Caucasians.

The UK **RDA** for infants is 7.5 µg. No dietary sources may be necessary for children and adults who are sufficiently exposed to sunlight, but during the winter children and adolescents who are still growing should receive 10 µg daily by supplementation. Adults with inadequate exposure to sunlight, such as the house-bound, may also need a supplement of 10 µg. In pregnancy and lactation, the RDA is 10 µg and this can only be achieved by supplementation (see APPENDIX II, SPECIAL NEEDS). Vitamin D deficiency results in soft or porous teeth and bones; this may lead to **rickets** in children and **osteomalacia** in adults as well as tooth decay. Vitamin D is the most toxic vitamin. A high intake (about 50 µg a day) can produce toxicity in infants, which causes loss of appetite, nausea, vomiting and poor growth. Adults are less susceptible to vitamin D toxicity, and only doses in excess of 250 µg a day cause the above symptoms.

vitamin E (also called **tocopherol**)   An **antioxidant**, vital for maintaining the structure of cell membranes. It also protects other vitamins such as vitamin A and vitamin C from oxidation. Vitamin E helps maintain low levels of **cholesterol** in the blood and keeps the blood thin, which helps prevent arterial blood clots and heart disease. It can help in the healing of burns and it may also be beneficial to those suffering from diseases that affect the nervous system, such as multiple sclerosis.

Vitamin E is found in wheat germ oil, vegetable oils, soya beans, leafy green vegetables, sunflower seeds, wholegrain cereals and polyunsaturated margarines. It is destroyed in some commercial methods of food processing, cooking and freezing; in the home, only the very high temperatures of deep frying destroy it. There is no UK **RDA**, but a daily dosage of about 0.3 µg is generally accepted as adequate for adults. Vitamin E deficiency due to low intake from the diet is very rare because of its wide distribution in foods and the small requirement. However, new-born babies may develop **anaemia** if their vitamin E intake is inadequate.

vitamin H   See **biotin**.

vitamin K   A vitamin essential to the production of several **proteins** including prothrombin, which is involved in blood clotting. It has been found to exist in three forms, one of which is obtained from food and the other two are synthesized within the body. Vitamin K_1, the form found in food, is present in broccoli, lettuce, cabbage, spinach, liver, alfalfa, safflower-seed oil, soya oil and kelp, and is stable to cooking and processing. The other two forms, K_2 and K_3, are synthesized by intestinal flora (microorganisms that live in the healthy gut). Antibiotics can indiscriminately destroy intestinal bacteria and eating live yoghurt, buttermilk and other dairy products may help to restore the natural gut flora. There is no **RDA**, but a daily intake of 100 µg is generally considered adequate for adults. Vitamin K deficiency is rare because K_2 and K_3 can be synthesized in the body. An absence of intestinal flora combined with a poor intake in the diet may cause haemorrhages and delayed blood clotting.

vitamin-enriched Foods to which manufacturers have added vitamins to supplement or increase quantities of those present naturally. In some cases enrichment is imposed legally; all margarines are required by law to contain added **vitamin A** and **D**. In these cases, foods are usually said to be fortified.

vodka An alcoholic drink of Russian origin. Vodka is usually made from cereals (especially rye) or potatoes. It usually contains 37.5% **alcohol** by volume. It has an energy value of 222 kcal/100 ml (or three measures), but is deficient in all other nutrients.

walnut The fruit of a deciduous tree of west Asian origin, with a hard, wrinkled shell and an oily, convoluted, two-lobed kernel. Walnuts are eaten whole and are added to cakes, pastries and salads to give flavour and texture. They have a high fat content, with a high proportion of **polyunsaturated fatty acids**, which can be extracted and used as edible oil. Walnuts also provide some **protein** (but they are not as good a source as most other nuts) and **dietary fibre**, small amounts of **starch** and **sugars**, and have an energy value of 525 kcal/100 g. Walnuts are rich in **potassium**, **manganese** and **phosphorus**, and they contain some **thiamin**, **vitamin B_6**, **folic acid** and **biotin**.

walnut oil The dark, fragrant oil extracted from the walnut. Walnut oil is used for seasoning. It is rich in **polyunsaturated fatty acid** and has an energy value of 899 kcal/100 g.

water Although essential for life, water is not considered a food or nutrient. About two-thirds of the body's weight is water, and almost all the body's processes inside and outside the cells require the presence of water. It comes into the body via food and drink and is also produced in the body during **metabolism**. Foods that provide the most water are milk, fruit and vegetables. It is lost in urine and faeces, through perspiration and breathing. A daily intake of 2 litres is usually sufficient to balance losses in healthy adults living in a climate such as the UK. If the balance is upset and water output exceeds input, due to excessive perspiration, diarrhoea or restricted intake, the body becomes dehydrated. In health, the body keeps a constant water balance so that if water intake is increased output is also increased because the kidneys excrete a more dilute urine. Water intoxication is rare and is usually associated with excess **sodium** loss rather than water intake.

water, drinking   The body needs a daily intake of at least 1 litre of water or beverages. Tap water contains varying amounts of minerals. Hard water contains significantly more calcium and other minerals than soft water. Hard water regions are associated with a lower risk of mortality from heart disease but the reason for this is as yet unknown. Calcium may have a protective function or there may be harmful substances in soft water. Soft water is more acidic and tends to dissolve lead and other unwanted trace elements out of pipes and containers. Tap water is treated and purified with a number of chemicals including large amounts of chlorine and fluorine. See also **mineral water**.

watercress   A leafy, green vegetable grown in running fresh water. Watercress is used in salads and as a garnish. It has a high water content and a low energy value of 14 kcal/100 g. It contains some **dietary fibre** and a small amount of **protein**; it is particularly rich in **vitamin A**, **folic acid**, **riboflavin** and **vitamin C**, and also provides reliable amounts of **potassium** and **calcium**.

watermelon The sweet-tasting, pink-fleshed fruit of an African melon plant. Watermelon has an exceptionally high water content, a small sugar content and a correspondingly low energy value of 21 kcal/100 g. It does not contain significant quantities of any **micronutrients** except for **pantothenic acid**.

weaning food See APPENDIX II, SPECIAL NEEDS.

wheat A cereal that represents a major source of **carbohydrate** and **protein** in the British diet. Wheat is chiefly used to make flour, and wheat flour is the main ingredient of bread. Wheat is also used in breakfast cereals and in making pasta. The wheat grain or seed is composed of the starchy endosperm, the bran layers and the germ. The **wholegrain** contains **protein**, **starch** and **dietary fibre**, and also provides **iron**, **calcium**, **niacin** and **thiamin**, and small amounts of **selenium**, **phosphorus**, **molybdenum** and **manganese**. Like other cereals it is deficient in vitamins A, C and B_{12}. Many of the micronutrients are seriously depleted in the making of white flour when the bran and germ are removed, but wholewheat flour retains the goodness of the natural wholegrain.

wheatbran The bran (fibrous outer husk) of wheat grains. Wheatbran is a rich source of **dietary fibre**, and this accounts for its beneficial effect on digestion. It adds bulk to the faeces and may be used in the treatment of constipation. It also provides **starch**, **protein**, some **fat** and reliable amounts of **potassium**, **phosphorus**, **niacin**, **folic acid** and **biotin**. Raw bran contains **phytic acid**, which interferes with the absorption of minerals such as calcium, iron, zinc and magnesium. To increase dietary fibre intake, it is therefore preferable to eat bran as an integral part of the wheat grain, as in wholemeal bread, pasta or wholegrain breakfast cereals. Wheatbran is removed during milling.

wheat germ The germ or embryo in the wheat grain or seed, situated at the lower end of the grain and consisting of the shoot and root. The germ is relatively rich in **protein**, and **fat** with a high proportion of **unsaturated fatty acids**. It is one of the best sources of **vitamin E** and the **B complex vitamins** as well as a good source of **iron**, **phosphorus**, **molybdenum**, **manganese** and **selenium**. It is liable to go rancid unless kept in a refrigerator. Processed germ is treated to prevent rancidity and virtually all the nutrients are retained.

wheat germ oil A highly nutritious **vegetable oil** derived from **wheat germ**. It is a rich source of **polyunsaturated fatty acids** (particularly **linoleic acid**) and has an energy value of 899 kcal/100 g. Wheat germ oil is used mainly as a dietary supplement rather than in cooking.

whisky A spirit made from fermented cereals (barley in Scotland and Ireland; rye or maize in the United States). The fermented grain is distilled and may be matured and/or blended. Whisky usually contains approximately 40% **alcohol** by volume. It has a high energy value of 222 kcal/100 g (three measures), but is deficient in all other nutrients.

whitebait Young fatty fish (usually herrings or sprats) that are coated in flour, fried and eaten whole. They have a very high **fat** content and a correspondingly high energy value of 525 kcal/100 g. They contain **protein** and are a good source of **calcium** (from the bones). They are also a good source of **iron**, but do not provide significant quantities of any vitamins once they have been subjected to the high temperatures used in frying.

whiting A white fish related to the cod and native to European seas. Whiting provides **protein**, only very small amounts of **fat** and has an energy value of 92 kcal/100 g when steamed. It contains some **potassium** and **sulphur**, but it is a poor source of **iron** when compared with fatty fish.

wholefoods Foods that have been refined or processed as little as possible and are eaten in their natural state, such as **wholegrain** or wholemeal flour. Wherever possible, none of the natural, nutritional properties of wholefoods have been removed, and nothing has been added too them. In many cases they have also been produced without using hormones, pesticides or fertilizers (to ensure that none of these substances have been used, look for foods labelled organic).

wholegrain (also called **wholemeal**) Grains of cereals that have not been refined in processing to remove any part of the grain. Most of the **B complex vitamins, fat, dietary fibre, iron, trace elements** and **vitamin E** are concentrated in the bran, germ and outer layers of the endosperm. The nutritional content of the cereal is reduced the more it is refined and these components are removed. Some of the nutrients may be partly replaced. White flour has iron, **thiamin, niacin** and **calcium** added by law, but it is still a comparatively poor source of fibre, vitamin E, and **pyridoxine**.

wholemeal See **wholegrain**.

wholewheat Wheat that has not been refined in processing. It contains all the nutrients present in the wholewheat grain, including the wheat bran, which is a good source of **dietary fibre**. See also **wholegrain**.

wine An alcoholic drink usually made by fermenting grapes (with water and sugar), although it may be made by fermenting many kinds of fruit or flower in this way. In grape wine, the grapes used may be black (red wines) or white (white wines) or both may be used (rosé wines). Varying amounts of sugar and water are added during the fermenting process to produce sweet, medium or dry wines. Sparkling wines may be produced by artificial carbonating or by secondary fermenting. The bubbles in champagne, a sparkling white wine, are achieved by a special secondary fermenting process. Most wines contain between 7.5 and 12.5% **alcohol** by volume. Sweet white wines and sparkling wines have the highest alcohol content. Sweet white wines have the highest sugar content and correspondingly higher energy values at 94 kcal/100 g. Red wines have the lowest sugar content; red wines and dry white wines have the lowest energy values at 66–68 kcal/100 g. Low alcohol and de-alcoholized wine is also available. Fortified wines (see **port** and **sherry**) have had extra alcohol or, in some cases, brandy added to them.

wine vinegar   Vinegar that has been made from wine. Either red or white wine may be used. Wine vinegar is often used in salad dressings because it has a more pleasant taste than malt vinegar.

winkles   Small molluscs (see **shellfish**). Winkles provide **protein** and only a very small amount of **fat** and have energy values of 74 kcal/100 g. They are usually cooked in sea water and therefore have a high **sodium** content. They also provide well-absorbed **iron** and **zinc** and are good sources of **calcium** and **magnesium**.

yam   The starchy tuber of any of a number of twining tropical plants. Yams have a high **starch**

content, provide a little **protein** and **dietary fibre** (including **pectin**) and a small amount of **sugar**. They have an energy content of 119 kcal/100 g (boiled yams), higher than potatoes, but contain less **B complex vitamins** and **vitamin C**.

yeast A substance consisting of single-celled fungi of the genus *Saccharomyces*, used in baking and brewing. The yeast used in baking is available in dried granules or as a cheesy culture. In warm, moist conditions (i.e. while dough is proving) it reproduces rapidly and releases carbon dioxide; this causes the dough to expand and rise. Yeast is used in brewing certain beers, because it ferments the sugars in the cereals used. Brewer's yeast is a rich source of some minerals and vitamins, especially **B complex vitamins** and is used as a dietary supplement. Yeast is also a natural inhabitant of the healthy digestive tract.

yeast infection A digestive or vaginal infection caused by excessive reproduction of intestinal yeast normally present in the healthy digestive tract. Accelerated reproduction may be promoted by a diet that is high in sugar, or it may be caused by long-term use of antibiotics, which have upset the normal balance of intestinal micoorganisms such as bacteria and fungi. Many symptoms of overpopulation with yeast or *Candida* have been reported, including diarrhoea, bloating and flatulence, headache or migraine, joint pains and fatigue. A medical diagnosis of *Candida* should be

273

made before treatment is started. Treatment initially is with a sugar-free diet.

yeast extract A savoury paste made by autolysis (self-digestion) of the cell walls of the yeast so that the contents are released. Yeast extract is used as a spread and may be added to soups and stew to add flavour. Yeast extract is a source of **B complex vitamins**, including **vitamin B$_{12}$**, and **protein**. It also provides **potassium**, **phosphorus** and **iron**. Spices and vegetable extract are added to concentrated yeast extract together with salt, which gives it a high **sodium** content. It is used in very small amounts and therefore has a negligible energy value.

yoghurt A milk product made by fermenting milk with bacteria (usually *Lactobacillus bulgaricus* and *Streptococcus thermophilus*) to produce **lactic acid** from the **lactose** in **milk**, that makes the milk curdle. Yoghurt can be made from whole milk, semi-skimmed milk and skimmed milk. Whole milk natural yoghurt has an energy value of 78 kcal/100 g, low fat natural yoghurt has an energy value of 53 kcal/100 g. It may have sugar, fruit or flavouring added to it. It is a good source of **protein**, **calcium** and **riboflavin**, and the low-fat varieties, made from skimmed or semi-skimmed milk, make useful alternatives to cream. The bacteria naturally present in yoghurt help to maintain the correct functioning of the digestive tract.

zinc A **trace element** that is an essential component of many **enzyme** systems. It is vital for growth and sexual maturation and it has a function in wound healing. Zinc is found in greatest amounts in milk, meat, liver, cheese, yoghurt, eggs, fish and shellfish (especially oysters). Nuts, vegetables, wholegrains and pulses also contain zinc, but it is not so well digested as from animal sources. There is no **RDA**, but a daily intake of 10 mg is considered adequate, an amount contained in the average UK diet. Zinc deficiency causes a degeneration in skin condition, slow healing of wounds and an increased susceptibilty to infections. It may cause a loss of sense of taste, loss of appetite, poor circulation, joint pains and general fatigue.

Appendix I

Losing and Gaining Weight

Losing Weight

At any one time, up to 60% of women and 30% of men are trying to lose weight, although by no means all are overweight. There has been a steady increase in the number of overweight people in the last fifty years and more infants and young children are also overweight than in previous decades.

Because much of the fat is found just below the skin, the degree of fatness can be assessed by skinfold thickness measurements using special callipers. However, the most common method of assessment is to compare body weight with height and body type. The acceptable weight range takes into account small, medium and heavy frames. A weight of 10% above the upper limit of the acceptable weight range is considered overweight and 20% above the upper limit is considered obese. However, perhaps the simplest method of determination of all is to take an honest look in a mirror, or to acknowledge the tightening waistbands or the bigger clothes size.

Fat accumulates in the body when more food is eaten than the body needs for maintenance and physical activity. In a small number of cases people eat to excess because of a physiological disturbance, but for the vast majority the reason is for the pleasure of eating. The overweight tend to eat more foods, particularly manufactured, processed foods, that have high fat and sugar contents. Over-indulgence in alcoholic drinks can also contribute to being overweight.

A person usually becomes overweight gradually over a period of months, even years. The supposed gains of 3–5 lbs after an over-indulgent weekend do not represent increases in body fat but of water. To gain one pound of fat you must consume 3500 kcal extra above your energy requirement.

The trigger that starts weight gain varies between individuals but common causes include a period of inactivity, giving up smoking, a period of stress, anxiety or depression, pregnancy and increasing age. The metabolism slows down with age, and the elderly may become less active but still eat the same amount of food as before.

The best way to prevent weight gain is to encourage sensible eating habits in young children. By laying down the foundations of a good diet early in life, the risks of overweight and obesity later can be reduced. Weight gain can be prevented by following the current recommendations for a balanced or prudent diet and taking some form of exercise regularly.

The numerous and varied cures and diets for overweight and obesity lead one to wonder whether they really do result in effective and long-term weight loss. The majority are aimed at small weight losses for special occasions. For more permanent weight loss there must be a lifelong alteration in eating habits and an increase in physical activity. The new diet must be nutritionally sound and pleasurable. Unfortunately the main problem is that it is the enjoyable high calorie foods that cause weight gain.

To reduce the degree of hardship, many aids have been launched onto the slimming market but none are substitutes for a long-term change in diet, and, at best, can only help in conjunction with a sensible, calorie-controlled diet. Anorectic drugs, diuretics and laxatives are not effective or safe methods of losing weight. A change in diet, usually in combination with some increase in physical activity, is so far the only proven method of effective weight loss.

Over the years, there have been a variety of diets claiming to be the ultimate answer to weight problems. The basis of all diets is that the energy entering the body from food and drink must be less than the body needs. If this happens, the body will go into a deficit (or negative balance), the body fat will be broken down and energy stores released to make up this deficit.

The most drastic form of weight loss is to go on a total fast. Initially, the glycogen stores in the body are used up and because this involves the rapid loss of water, there is a very encouraging immediate weight loss. This does not continue, however, because the body soon switches to its store of body fat to make up the energy supply.

This causes the body to produce substances called ketone bodies, which can accumulate in the blood, resulting in headaches, nausea and an unpleasant smell of acetone (like nail polish remover) on the breath. In some people, fasting can change the rhythm of the heart. Fasting is a method of weight loss that should only be undertaken under strict medical and dietetic supervision. The aim of any diet is to break down body fat, and on sensible reducing diets this can be done without the production of ketone bodies.

There have been many popular diets over the years, but few seem to stand the test of time.

The *Eat Fat and Grow Slim* diet is comprised mainly of foods high in fat and protein, plus fruit and vegetables. Milk is restricted but the use of cream is positively encouraged. The high fat intake may make you feel full but this diet certainly does not follow the current recommendations for a balanced, healthy diet.

In the *Low Carbohydrate Diet*, the carbohydrate is limited and rather than counting calories, you count carbohydrate units. This type of diet goes against the accepted view that we should be eating more bread, pasta, rice and potatoes and less meat and dairy products.

The *Atkins Diet* permits a wide range of foods but severely restricts carbohydrate, to the point where ketone bodies are produced.

The *Scarsdale Diet* has a high protein content, contains very little (if any) fat and a reduced carbohydrate content. There is no portion control. It lacks certain essential nutrients and the high protein intake is both unnecessary and expensive.

In the *Pritkin Diet*, the level of dietary fibre is high but low in calories, and the restrictions on protein and fat are very drastic. The diet is very monotonous because only a limited range of foods is permitted.

The *F Plan Diet* is a low-calorie, high dietary fibre diet with the emphasis on eating a wide range of cereals, fruit and vegetables. The sudden increase in fibre intake may lead to discomfort from wind and diarrhoea but this diet comes closest to the current recommendations for a balanced diet.

Very Low Calorie Diets are the most controversial of the formula diets. In the initial weeks, food is replaced by a formula drink that provides all the daily requirements of vitamins and minerals but with only 400–500 kcal. These drinks may have a use in treating the grossly obese, under medical and dietetic supervision, but are not recommended for the mildly overweight.

The basis for all treatments is to reduce the energy intake and the most common, most successful method is the low-calorie diet. Such diets allow unlimited amounts of some vegetables and fruits, and clear drinks, i.e. those items that contain very few calories. Foods that contain moderate amounts of energy but are good sources of essential nutrients, such as meat, fish, eggs, potatoes, bread and milk are allowed in weighed amounts. Fats and sugar, and those foods that contain them, are avoided completely. For many people who only need to lose a little weight or to maintain an acceptable weight, the current recommendations of eating less fat and sugar and more starchy carbohydrate foods rich in dietary fibre are sufficient, as long as attention is paid to portion size.

Eating Less Fat Most of the fat in our diet comes from meat and meat products, spreading fats (e.g. margarine and butter), milk and milk products and cooking fats (e.g. oil and lard). It is also present in cakes, biscuits, pastry and chocolate. It is possible to considerably reduce the fat intake by making the following changes: **1.** Choose lean cuts of meat. **2.** Trim off any visible fat from meat, such as chops or steak. **3.** Drain off excess fat from casseroles and mince dishes. **4.** Use pulses to extend meat dishes so that you actually have smaller portions of meat and at the same time increase your intake of complex or starchy carbohydrates. **5.** Eat more fish and poultry, but avoid the poultry skin because the fat is just underneath, and drain off any oil from canned fish. Alternatively buy fish canned in brine. **6.** Grill, steam or microwave rather than fry. **7.** Buy skimmed or semi-skimmed milk instead of whole milk. **8.** Buy low-fat or reduced-fat varieties of cheese. **9.** Use a low-fat spread instead of butter or margarine, and use it sparingly. **10.** Cut bread

thicker so that you will spread proportionitely
less fat. **11.** Use low-fat natural yoghurt or *fromage frais* instead of cream, mayonnaise or
sauces. **12.** Do not allow fats to crowd out the
important starchy carbohydrate foods such as
bread, cereals, pulses, vegetables and fruit. **13.**
Always buy a low-fat alternative if one is
available.

Eating Less Sugar Sugar in the diet comes from
ordinary table sugar added to hot drinks, breakfast cereals and fruit, but also from chocolate,
sweets, soft drinks and, of course, sweet-tasting
food such as cakes and biscuits. Anyone trying to
lose weight should be looking carefully at the
amount of sugar they consume. The level of sugar
intake can be reduced by following these suggestions: **1.** Reduce and eventually cut out all
table sugar from drinks, breakfast cereals and any
sprinkled on fruit, etc. **2.** Eat more fresh fruit
instead of sweet puddings. **3.** Buy canned fruit in
natural juice rather than in heavy syrup. **4.** Cut
out sweets, chocolate, soft drinks, cakes and biscuits. Pure fruit juice, mineral water and soda
water are good alternatives to sweet drinks,
although even fruit juices contain natural sugar
and therefore some calories. Oatcakes, scones and
currant bread contain less sugar than other cakes
and biscuits, and there are many more sugar-
reduced products such as jam, breakfast cereal
and yoghurt available in shops and supermarkets.

Eating more Starch and Fibre Having cut down

your intake of fat and sugar, you must increase
your intake of starchy or complex carbohydrates.
Such foods are a far less concentrated source of
calories than fat-containing foods. The bulkiness
of starchy foods makes it difficult to eat excessive
amounts of them, unlike sugar and sugar-
containing foods. Complex carbohydrate foods
such as cereals, pulses, fruit and vegetables all
make significant contributions to the intake of
nutrients and micronutrients. Following this list
of suggestions will help to increase the amount of
starch and fibre: 1. Switch to wholemeal bread,
rolls and pitta bread. 2. Use wholegrain breakfast
cereals, avoiding those with added sugar. 3. Use
half wholemeal and half white flour in cooking. 4.
Use brown rice and wholemeal pasta. 5. Eat potatoes in their skins, either baked or boiled. 6. Prepare more dishes that are based on rice, pasta,
beans, potatoes and vegetables. 7. High fibre
foods absorb more water in your body and as you
increase your fibre intake you will need to drink
more fluid. A well-planned diet, or, better, a
longterm healthy eating programme, should
result in a steady loss of 2 lb a week after a possible
initial larger loss. There should be no tiredness (as
frequently experienced on severely calorie-
restricted diets) and you should be able to carry on
normal daily activities quite happily.

Some Self-help Measures First check with the
acceptable weight tables that you do need to lose

weight. It is also advisable to discuss your diet with your doctor first.

Keep a diary of your eating and drinking habits for a few days before you start dieting. You will then be able to find out more about your eating habits and perhaps what has caused you to overeat. You may discover that you are a night-eater, that you are addicted to certain foods, that you prefer eating snacks rather than meals or even that you eat most of your food standing up.

Work out what your motivation to lose weight is – for looks or health, because you are tired or breathless or because you already suffer from complications associated with overweight or obesity. Set yourself targets, including immediate ones, otherwise the final goal may seem too daunting. Weigh yourself regularly once a week on the same scales, at the same time, wearing the same clothes (or nothing). If you find calorie counting helpful, there are several useful publications, especially the *Collins Gem Calorie Counter*. Group therapy in the form of a slimming club is a great help to some people and there are several networks throughout the country.

Exercise must also become a regular part of your life. It pushes up the energy output and, contrary to popular belief, it does not increase the appetite; in fact, the regulating mechanism in the brain seems to work better at increased levels of activity.

Gaining Weight

It is a common observation that some people eat whatever and whenever they want without gaining weight. Thin people seem able to increase the energy needed for self-maintenance and so they can burn off any excess dietary intake rather than storing it as body fat. Thus, for some people, gaining weight is not an easy task, particularly as any weight gain should be mainly from an increase in muscle mass or lean tissue rather than from body fat. In a normally healthy, but thin person, gains in muscle mass are the result of regular training and a correct diet. Your diet should be well-balanced and high in starchy carbohydrate, plenty of wholemeal cereals (bread, pasta and rice) plus fresh fruit and vegetables (including potatoes) and pulses (beans, peas and lentils).

Eating patterns are also important; try not to miss meals, cultivate a regular meal pattern and aim for three meals a day, including breakfast. Eat sensible snacks between meals such as milky drinks, sandwiches, dried fruit and nuts and muesli bars. Increase your portion sizes and have at least two, if not three, courses at each meal.

We are not all meant to be the same height and weight and if you are healthy and eating a balanced diet with average portion sizes, you should perhaps accept that you are your 'ideal' weight.

Acceptable Weight Range

Height (m)	Men (kg)	Women (kg)
1.45	.....	42-53
1.48	.....	42-54
1.50	.....	43-55
1.52	.....	44-57
1.54	.....	44-58
1.56	.....	45-58
1.58	54-64	46-59
1.60	52-65	48-61
1.62	53-66	49-62
1.64	54-67	50-64
1.66	55-69	51-65
1.68	56-71	52-66
1.70	58-73	53-67
1.72	59-74	55-69
1.74	60-75	56-70
1.76	62-77	58-72
1.78	64-79	59-74
1.80	65-80	.....
1.82	66-82	.....
1.84	67-84	.....
1.86	69-86	.....
1.88	71-88	.....
1.90	73-90	.....
1.92	75-93	.....

Appendix II

Special Needs

Pregnancy

As soon as you want to start a family, it is a good idea to think about your diet. If you are underweight, you should try to gain some weight because this will improve your chances of getting pregnant. Once pregnant, the most vulnerable stage for the developing foetus is the first few weeks, precisely the time when you may not know that you are pregnant, so aim for a healthy diet from the moment you decide to conceive.

Excessive drinking can lead to foetal alcohol syndrome, which causes mental and physical retardation in the baby. The effects of moderate consumption of alcohol are not yet fully known and the best approach would be to avoid alcohol pre- and peri-conceptually.

During pregnancy, the rapid growth of the foetus makes increased nutritional demands on the mother. The body adapts to this greater demand by increasing the absorption and decreasing the excretion of nutrients, and the metabolism generally becomes more efficient, but changes should also be made to the diet. The total energy cost of pregnancy is about 84 000 kcal, 100 kcal extra a day during the first quarter, and 300–400 kcal extra a day during the remainder of the pregnancy. In fact, an average increase in intake of 250 kcal per day is usually enough, the remainder being made up by a decrease in activity and therefore energy requirement.

A good guide to how much you need to increase your energy intake is your weight gain. If the rate of gain is acceptable, you can assume your intake is adequate and you just need to concentrate on the variety of foods to ensure an adequate intake of essential nutrients.

Iron requirements are increased even though there are no losses due to menstruation. If the iron intake level before pregnancy was adequate, the body's reserves and the increased absorption that comes with pregnancy will meet the requirements without the need to increase the dietary intake. If you start the pregnancy with poor iron stores, the low reserves and low intake may lead to iron deficiency anaemia, and a supplement will be necessary to correct the deficiency. In general it is a good idea to eat meat regularly and to get an adequate intake of vitamin C from fruit and vegetables, which help in the absorption of iron.

Calcium requirements are increased during pregnancy, but so is absorption. However, the efficiency of calcium absorption is impaired if the diet contains a lot of fibre, and you should ensure that you eat foods that are good sources of calcium every day. Sufficient vitamin intake should be assured by a diet that contains plenty of variety, but it is worth paying attention to your intake of vitamin D, C and folic acid.

If you start your pregnancy around your acceptable body weight for height, you should aim to gain about 9 kg, if you start overweight you should gain about 7.5 kg and if you start underweight you should gain about 13.5kg. This is true weight gain and does not include any gain caused by fluid retention.

There are several nutrition-related problems that can occur during pregnancy. Nausea and vomiting (including morning sickness) can be alleviated by eating carbohydrate-rich foods at regular intervals, such as toast and jam, sandwiches, plain biscuits and breakfast cereals. Rest, fresh air and avoidance of long journeys may also help.

Heartburn is another common complaint and can be eased by eating small, frequent snacks (particularly of milk and yoghurt) and by avoiding spicy and fatty foods, carbonated drinks, citrus fruit and fruit juices.

Constipation may be caused by iron supplements that have been prescribed and you should tell your doctor if this occurs; otherwise try to include plenty of foods rich in dietary fibre and keep up a good intake of fluids.

Lactation

If you have been eating a normal and varied diet throughout your pregnancy, and have been following the general healthy eating principles, you should just eat and drink more to satisfy your hunger and thirst. The energy cost of lactation is quite considerable, up to 500 kcal extra a day. The larger the baby, the bigger the demand that will be made on your milk supply and the greater will be your appetite. If you limit your intake it can cause tiredness and eventually will affect the milk supply. Increases in protein requirements are normally met by a balanced diet that provides sufficient energy. Although there are no specific requirements for fat and carbohydrate, these will need to be increased to meet the greater energy demands. Dietary fibre intake should be high, especially if you experience constipation. A good intake of fluid is vital for milk production but it is wise to avoid excessive intakes of strong tea, coffee and alcohol. If your diet is varied and supplying enough energy, vitamin and mineral intakes should also be adequate. Few lactating women need to take a supplement.

It is important to establish a regular eating pattern, to avoid any slimming while you continue to feed your baby, and to include variety in your diet and to drink when thirsty and eat when hungry.

Infants and Young Children

The best start you can give your baby is to breast-feed. It provides all the nutrients necessary, protects against infection and helps the emotional bonding between mother and baby. Breast-milk is less likely to cause allergic reactions than other milks. It is always readily available at the correct concentration and temperature. Breast-feeding also helps you to loose body fat and return to your pre-pregnancy weight. It is also economical – it costs less to feed the lactating mother than it does to bottle-feed.

On the negative side, breast-feeding also makes demands on the mother. It is not always easy to establish and keep up an adequate milk supply and there is no reassurance of how much your baby is taking at each feed. It can cause embarrassment and jealousy in the family, and can make it difficult for you to return to work.

There are some situations in which breast-feeding is not the best method; if the mother needs to have regular drug therapy, if either the mother or the baby have physical problems, or if the baby has a low birth weight, is ill or is going to be adopted.

If the mother's diet is adequate, the breast-milk will supply all the energy and essential nutrients that the new baby needs. However, when the baby is one month old, it is advisable to give him or her vitamin drops. These are specially formulated for babies and are available from your local clinic, health centre or chemist.

The alternative to breast-feeding is bottle-feeding using an infant milk formula, manufactured from cows' milk or soya milk. Although these formulae are not exactly the same as breast-milk in composition, their nutrient content is much closer to breast-milk than the milks that were produced 20 years ago. Manufacturers follow guidelines for composition laid down by the Department of Health. If you intend to bottle-feed your baby, your health visitor or midwife will help you decide which formula to use. It is very important that you prepare each feed according to the manufacturer's instructions on the package. Errors in reconstitution can lead to a feed that is too concentrated or too dilute for your baby.

Milk is a particularly good breeding ground for bacteria and strict hygiene is required when making up feeds. Vitamins and minerals are already added to the infant milk formula and extra supplements are not usually needed at first. It is important to keep a check on the fluid intake of your baby. As a general guide, a young baby usually needs about 150 ml per kg of fluid per day. Progress can be monitored by growth rate and how contented your baby seems (a baby will suck until his or her thirst and hunger are satisfied).

Weaning is the gradual process of replacing breast or bottle-feeding with a mixed diet. The whole process can take at least six months and during this time your baby will develop the ability to chew and bite. Weaning usually starts between 3 and 8 months. A baby who is still hungry after a good feed is probably ready to be weaned. At this stage, milk alone cannot supply all the nutrients. Certainly by 6 months, the iron stores laid down in the baby before birth are used up. Milk is not a good source of iron and so other iron-containing foods must be introduced. Your baby will also be physically unable to drink the volume of milk needed to meet the increased energy requirements.

In the initial stages of weaning, the nutrient content of the foods offered are not as important as the consistency (which should be thin and smooth) and the taste (which should be mild or neutral). Foods should be introduced one at a time so that if your baby reacts in any way, you know which food to avoid. Usual first foods include baby rice, cooked and pureed fruits and vegetables and manufactured baby foods.

Over the next few months you should gradually introduce more foods, and gradually change the consistency so that it is more lumpy, until your baby (usually by about one year) can manage chopped family meals.

The Department of Health recommends that vitamin supplements should be given to infants and young children aged from 6 months up to at least 2 years and preferably 5 years, although some breast-fed babies will have been given vitamin drops since they were one month old. No salt or sugar should be added to the weaning baby's food. A continued intake of breast milk or of an infant milk formula throughout the first year is generally recommended.

The pre-school child is still dependent on others for food. As wide a variety of foods as possible should be offered, which are enjoyable and can be easily managed either with utensils or fingers. Small children are not able to eat large amounts of food at infrequent intervals and should be given smaller meals with regular nutritious snacks in between. Food fads and fussiness are very common in the pre-school child and although it is hard, you should never let eating problems become an issue or mealtimes a battleground.

Current general guidelines for healthy eating are not totally applicable to the pre-school child but you can gradually introduce healthy eating habits, especially if the rest of the family are following them. Young children need a moderate intake of fat, otherwise the diet becomes too bulky. They stop eating when they feel full, but before they have actually eaten enough to meet their energy requirements. A moderate fat intake can be achieved by cutting off any visible fat, using more lean meat, poultry and fish and using a margarine with a high proportion of polyunsaturated fatty acids. Milk and milk products are a staple dietary item until at least five years of age. Skimmed and semi-skimmed milk are not usually recommended because of their low energy value and poor vitamin A content. From the age of two, semi-skimmed milk can be introduced (especially if the rest of the family is using it), as long as the overall dietary intake from other sources provides sufficient energy and fat soluble vitamins. Fully skimmed milk is not recommended for any child under the age of five.

Too much fibre can make the diet too bulky, especially for a young child who does not have a large appetite. It is sometimes a good idea to offer high fibre foods as snacks rather than at meals. Sugar and salt intake should be kept to a minimum.

The Elderly

The overall message is to enjoy your food and make sure it contains all the essential nutrients for health. Some of the current guidelines are too restrictive for the elderly, because they deal with excesses in the diet, whereas the problems of the elderly are more to do with loss of appetite and interest in food. The diet must provide sufficient energy to maintain body weight, because a diet low in energy is likely to be low in essential nutrients. Poor exposure to sunlight may lead to a lack of vitamin D. If it is not possible to go out, then rich sources of vitamin D must be supplied in the diet, such as margarine, fish paté and soft canned fish.

Constipation is a common complaint, and fibre intake should be increased gradually to avoid any bowel discomfort. At the same time, more fluids should be drunk. Unfortunately, elderly people often loose their sense of thirst, so it may be necessary to make a conscious effort to drink.

Vegetarian, Vegan and Macrobiotic Diets

The term 'vegetarian' covers many different eating habits. Lacto-vegetarians eat all plant foods together with dairy foods, such as milk, cheese and yoghurt, and ovo-lacto-vegetarians also include eggs.

Vegans eat no animal foods, only foods of plant origin and the most restricted diets of all are the macrobiotic and fruitarian diets. Many people are becoming part-time or demi-vegetarians for health reasons. They are eating less red meat and more poultry and fish than they used to, and some are lacto-vegetarians at home, only eating meat when they are away from home.

The reasons for becoming a vegetarian are many. Some adopt these eating habits for health reasons, others for ecological reasons (on a pro rata basis it takes more land to produce animal foods than plant foods). Others are concerned that because animals are so high up the food chain, they will contain greater concentrations of pollutants (the aftereffects of the nuclear reactor explosion at Chernobyl are an example of this type of concern). Religious and ethical reasons, such as cruelty to animals, are other powerful reasons for becoming a vegetarian.

Although the lacto-vegetarian may have a high intake of fat, and particularly fat with a high proportion of saturated fatty acids, most vegetarians tend to have low fat intakes and increased dietary fibre intakes. Indeed research shows that vegetarians tend to have lower blood cholesterol levels and body weights, both factors that help to protect the body against heart disease. The high fibre intake also protects against certain diseases of the bowel. Vegetarian diets can therefore be as healthy, if not healthier, than some diets that contain meat. However, becoming a vegetarian does not simply mean cutting out meat or all animal products. The diet must be made up of foods that will provide those nutrients that animal products would otherwise offer. The more restricted the diet becomes, the harder and more important it is to understand how to maintain a balanced diet that provides all the essential nutrients.

Vegetarians need to make as wide as possible a choice from the following groups of food: **1.** All cereals and starchy vegetables, including bread, pasta, rice, breakfast cereals, oats and potatoes. **2.** Fruit, vegetables and fruit and vegetable juices. **3.** Milk, yoghurt and cheese – from cows' or soya milk. **4.** Eggs, pulses (peas, beans and lentils), nuts and seeds. **5.** Vegetable oil and vegetable margarine. Lacto-vegetarians and ovo-lacto-vegetarians generally have no problem in eating enough food to meet their energy and nutrient requirements. Iron is perhaps the only nutrient that may be lacking because meat is usually the main source of this mineral in the diet. Vegetarians obtain their iron from pulses, nuts and dried fruit and wholegrain cereals. By including foods rich in vitamin C (such as fresh fruit and vegetables) at the same meal or as snacks, the absorption of iron can be increased.

The vegan diet is a bulkier diet and it is harder, even impossible in some cases, for young children to manage to eat sufficient to meet their energy requirements before they feel full. Many adults also find it bulky, but learn to adapt with time. Protein is not usually a cause for concern in a vegan diet, provided that the diet contains a mixture of cereals, pulses, nuts and seeds. Such a variety provides all the essential amino acids that are required by the body. The most likely nutrients and micronutrients to cause problems are calcium, vitamin D and Vitamin B_{12}.

Dairy products are usually the main source of calcium, and vegans must ensure that their diet includes plenty of nuts, soya products and dark green vegetables. Sesame seeds (and tahini which is made from them) are particularly rich sources of calcium. Vitamin D should be obtained in sufficient amounts from the action of sunlight on the skin and this can be topped-up with a dietary source of fortified margarine. Vitamin B_{12} is not naturally present in a vegan diet as it is found almost exclusively in animal foods. The exceptions are miso, tempeh, baker's and brewer's yeast extracts and fortified foods such as some soya milks. If these foods are not included regularly, a supplement of vitamin B_{12} is needed. Again, because vegetable sources of iron are poorly absorbed, there must be a frequent consumption of pulses, wholegrains, dried fruit, nuts and dark green leafy vegetables together with foods rich in vitamin C.

In a macrobiotic diet all foods are divided up on the Chinese principles of Yin and Yang. Typical Yin foods are acidic and contain potassium and sugars, such as fruit, typical Yang foods are alkaline and contain sodium, such as cereals. The perfect balance of Yin and Yang is to be found in brown rice and this is the ultimate goal, or level, of the macrobiotic diet. This is reached by going through seven levels, giving up meat, fruit and vegetables at various stages. Such a diet, particularly at the final levels, can lead to malnutrition, anaemia and vitamin deficiencies. Fruitarian diets are made up solely of fruit, nuts and seeds and are not balanced diets.

Athletes

Athletes tend to pay more attention to vitamin and mineral supplements than to the more important task of providing the body with energy and fluid. When exercising hard and regularly, it is important to eat sufficient amounts of carbohydrate to maintain the stores of glycogen in the muscles. You must also drink plenty of fluid to prevent the body becoming dehydrated through sweating.

The body has a vast source of potential energy stored in body fat (even in the leanest of athletes) but its conversion to energy is slow. Carbohydrate, in the form of glycogen stored in the muscles and liver, supplies energy at the much faster rate required to meet the immediate demands of exercise. Whatever the exercise, duration and intensity, carbohydrate will be used, together with fat, but it is carbohydrate that is the limiting fuel. Only the glycogen in the actual exercising muscles can be used and it is therefore important that these stores are restocked after every bout of exercise. It is also why training programmes should be designed to use different sets of muscles, for instance, mixing running with weight training. If the muscle glycogen stores are not restocked after each exercise session, you will have less and less available 'fast fuel'. Incomplete refuelling over successive days leads to fatigue and heavy muscles, and performance will suffer.

To keep up the level of muscle glycogen, you should eat a diet high in carbohydrate, with 50–60% of the total energy coming solely from carbohydrate. Fat intake should be kept down and, contrary to popular belief, you do not need a high protein intake. A normal diet that provides sufficient energy will also provide enough protein. The increase in muscle comes from training and a diet high in carbohydrate, so allowing training to take place at high intensity, and not from a high protein intake. An athlete's diet is therefore not unlike that being recommended generally, the same dietary message applies to eating for performance and eating for health. However, because of the often much higher energy requirement of athletes, a proportion of the carbohydrate intake may have to come from simple sugars, otherwise the diet may be too bulky.

Before competition, glycogen stores should be well-stocked. Athletes taking part in endurance events such as a marathon, or those involved in a competition lasting several days often increase their intake of carbohydrate even more just before the event and they reduce their training programme. This has the effect of increasing the glycogen content in the muscles even more. The disadvantage of such a procedure is that the increased glycogen is associated with an increase in water retention. The excess body weight that this causes should be taken into consideration, particularly if your sport involves you making a specific, competitive weight. Your precompetition meal should be carbohydrate in content, easily digested and probably not eaten less than 2–3 hours before you start, although there is considerable individual variation in the optimum timing.

The temperature of the body is controlled between very fine limits. During exercise, heat is produced, which, if unchecked would cause a potentially dangerous rise in body temperature. The mechanism of sweating is very effective in bringing the temperature under control, but in so doing the body loses vital fluid together with some electrolytes. The electrolyte loss is not important in most situations because a much greater proportion of water is lost, so that the remaining body electrolytes are more concentrated. Fluid can be replaced by drinking plain water. Sports drinks are available and although they make claims about their carbohydrate and electrolyte contents, these are added primarily to help the absorption of water.

To avoid dehydration during exercise, you should always start fully hydrated, and have a drink up to 30 minutes before you begin exercising. It is very important to drink little and often during exercise and not wait until you feel thirsty, particularly during long exercise sessions, or in very hot weather. Once you stop exercising replace fluids with a drink (non-alcoholic) as soon as you can.

Athletes do not need extra vitamins and minerals above those that are contained in a good balanced diet that is meeting the increased energy requirement of the athlete. Athletes who are eating a poor diet, especially those who are limiting their food intake to keep to a particular weight such as jockeys, ballet dancers, gymnasts and lightweight rowers, may not be getting sufficient vitamins and minerals. Ideally the diet should be corrected, but this is not always possible or realistic, in which case a supplement should be taken regularly. Increasing the vitamin and mineral intake to an acceptable level may well have a beneficial effect on athletic performance but further increasing an otherwise adequate level will not affect performance at all.